BEST BOOKS FOR
YOGA
LOVERS

Graphic Design

Mattias Långström

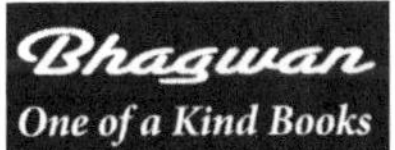

BEST BOOKS FOR
YOGA
LOVERS

Index

PATANJALI YOGA SÛTRAS

TO BE PRESENT IN YOGA

Translation and comments

Jan Fahleman

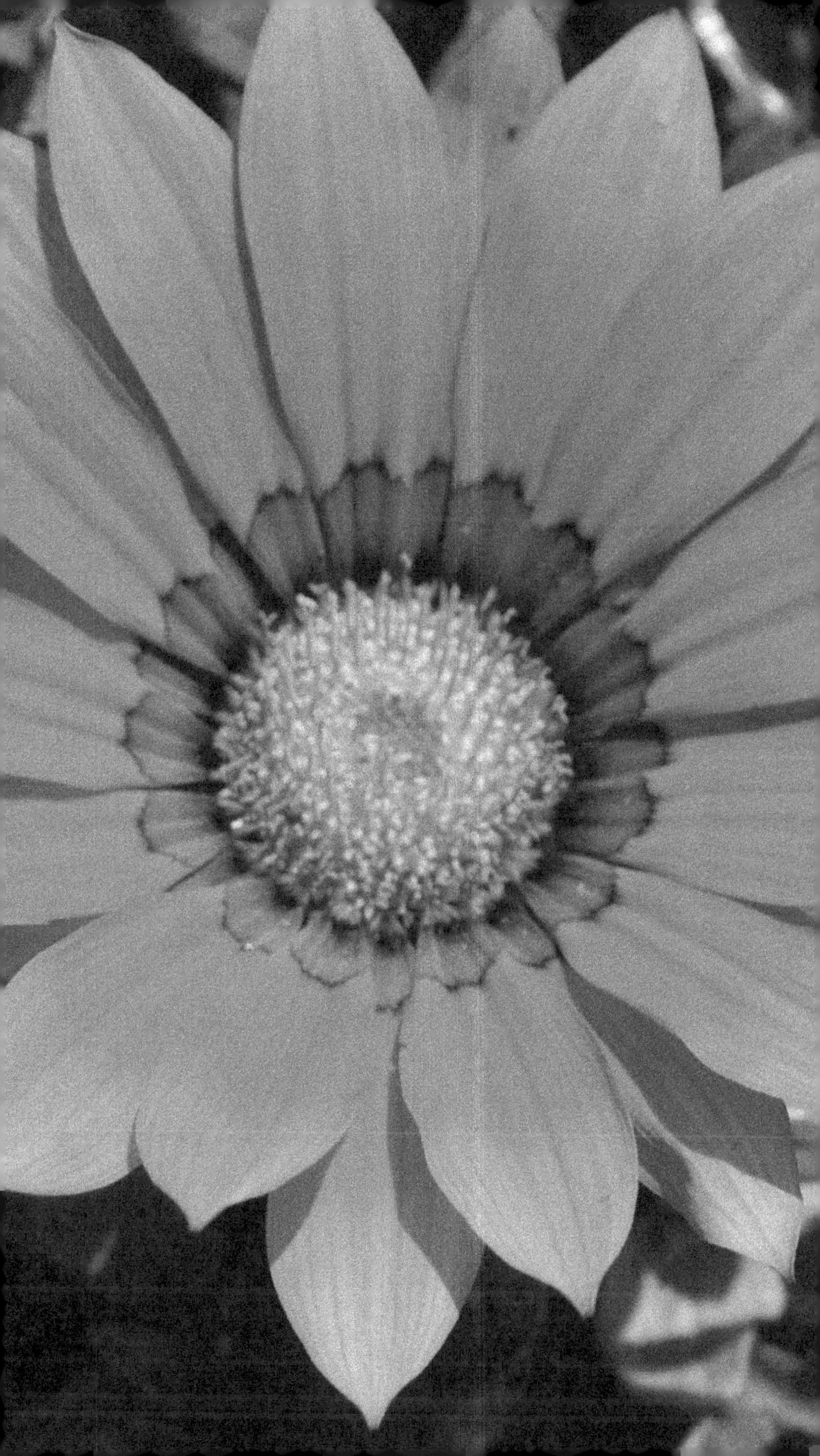

Introduction

Yoga Sutras by Patanjali has achieved the status of being one of the most important classical yoga texts and Patanjali's definition of yoga is also one of the most widespread. He was the first to methodically record the ancient and timeless knowledge of yoga in eight classical steps. With Patanjali, yoga was incorporated into the Hindu tradition as one of six philosophical paths and gained its distinct Indian character.

A good way to approach the knowledge is to read a few sutras at a time. They are logical in their structure and you will slowly understand more and more.

Patanjali's classic sutras are carefully interpreted by the Swedish author Jan Fahleman. He has practiced meditation and yoga asanas for many decades and applied some of Patanjali's sutras. He has studied Vedic literature and various spiritual masters since the 1970s.

Preface

Patañjali lived about 200 years B.C. in India. There is little historical information about him. He has often been called Maharishi Patañjali. In his work "Yoga Sutras" he explained and described yoga with 196 short sutras. These sutras can be seen as formulas or aphorisms of philosophical wisdom. They were originally not written down but were passed on orally from teacher to student.

The word Yoga can be derived from the Sanskrit word yuj which means union and refers to union with the divine. This compound is not an event that will happen in the future, it occurs in the present, but the individual must be aware of this relationship. Patañjali describes in his sutras how the obstacles to this awareness can be bridged. He gives instructions on eight paths for practical application. Patanjali's theoretical philosophy can be verified by experience through practical application.

Unfortunately, there are many of misconceptions when it comes to yoga. The prevailing view is that yoga is mostly different postures called asanas. Patanjali explains that Yoga asanas is but one of the eight paths that can lead to the state of Consciousness called yoga or Samādhi.

I have chosen to write simply and understandably, with expressions and terms that many spiritual teachers use today. My starting point was Patanjali's original text in Sanskrit, but in my comments also draw from my own personal experience of yoga. I have written comments where I experienced the need for a clarification and have tried to keep these comments as brief as possible.

Throughout, the Sanskrit and the transliterated texts are on the left page and the english translation is on the right side one.

Jan Fahleman
Stockholm 2021

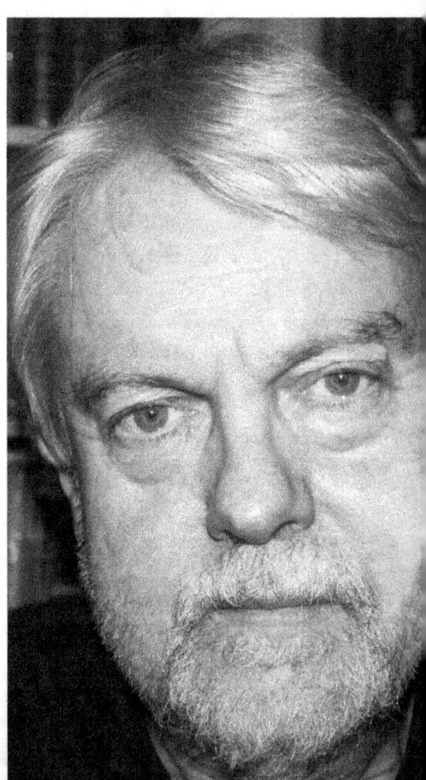

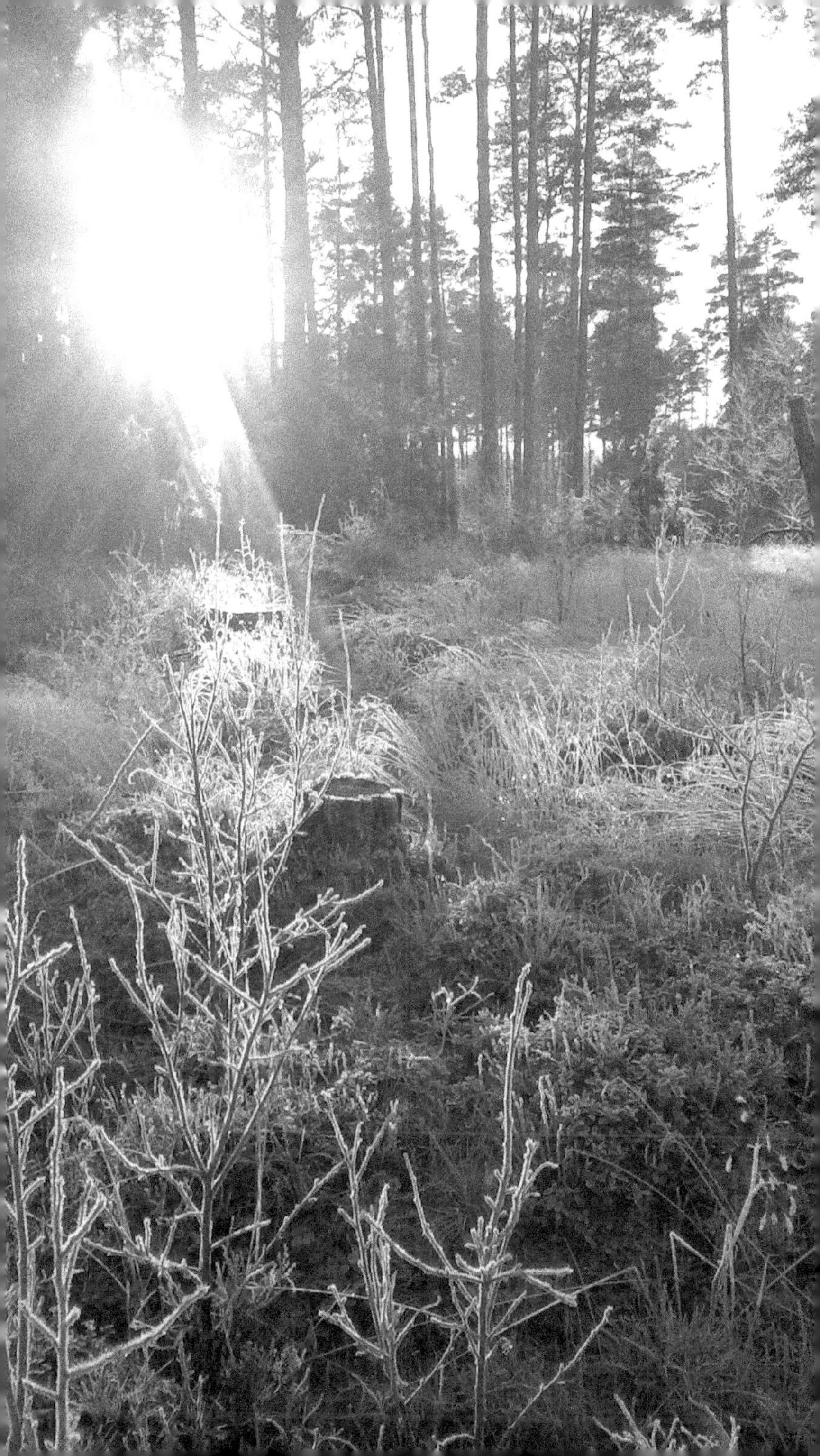

Chapter 1

SAMĀDHI PĀDA

About the state of awareness named

Samādhi

अथ योगानुशासनम्॥१॥

1. Atha yogānuśāsanam

योगश्चित्तवृत्तनिरोधः॥२॥

2. Yogaś citta vṛtti nirodhaḥ

तदा द्रष्टुः स्वरूपेऽवस्थानम्॥३॥

3. Tadā draṣṭuḥ svarūpe'vasthānam

वृत्तसिारूप्यमतिरत्र॥४॥

4. Vṛtti sārūpyam itaratra

वृत्तयः पञ्चतय्यः क्लष्टिा अक्लष्टिाः॥५॥1

5. Vṛttayaḥ pañcatayyaḥ kliṣṭā akliṣṭāḥ

1. Here begins the exposition of Yoga.

2. Yoga arises when awareness is no longer bound by the mind.

To be in the state of "Yoga", requires that the senses ie. thoughts, emotions and objects are not obstacles. The sense perceptions may continue to exist, but awareness is no longer bound by them in the state of yoga.

(Awareness is the individual focus and presence that provides experiences in the present).

3. Then the seer is aware of itself.

When the seer is aware of the Self, ie. is present in Consciousness, the true identity is revealed. The identity created by the mind is then seen as false, unreal and created out of ignorance.

(Consciousness is the absolute pure cosmic Consciousness that has many names: God, the Holy Spirit, the Spirit, Self, Being, Tao, or Brahman. Few words have so many prejudices and definitions as the word God. God is often referenced to a being in the outer life that one is separated from. Therefore Consciousness a better word in this context.)

4. Otherwise Consciousness is identified with the sensations.

Merely being aware of mental activity and sensory objects implies a limitation in experience of life. Obviously, it's good to be able to be present in the mind, but it may prevent the presence of Consciousness.

5. There are five different state of mind, some creates suffering while others do not.

In the relative changing life there is both happiness and suffering. As long as awareness is tied to the mind, both suffering and happiness will be experienced.

परमाणवपिर्ययवकिल्पनिद्रास्मृतयः॥६॥

6. Pramāṇa viparyaya vikalpa nidrā smṛtayaḥ

परत्यक्षानुमानागमाः परमाणानि॥७॥

7. Pratyakṣānumānāgamāḥ pramāṇāni

वपिर्ययो मथिया्ज्ञानमतदरूपप्रतष्ठिम्॥८॥

8. Viparyayo mithyā-jñānam atad-rūpa pratiṣṭham

शब्दज्ञानानुपाती वस्तुशून्यो वकिल्पः॥९॥

9. Śabda-jñānānupātī vastu-śūnyo vikalpaḥ

अभावप्रत्ययालम्बना वृत्तिर्निद्रा॥१०॥

10. Abhā-vapratyayālambanā vṛttir nidrā

6. They are; (pramana) valid knowledge (viparyaya) ignorance, (vikalpa) illusion (nidra) sleep and (smrti) memory.

7. Valid knowledge (pramana) is obtained by direct experience, by drawing conclusions and by external testimony.

This knowledge is obtained through the sense organs and by the intellect, which draws conclusions and by information coming from the environment. This is relative knowledge which the mind handles.

8. Ignorance (viparyaya) arises from misinterpretation of what is experienced.

The mind often wants to interpret what is perceived to fit with the situation that the mind is experiencing. This experience is often related to the past but also to an anticipated future, but it's not always this interpretation is consistent with the reality of the present.

9. Illusion (vikalpa) is to imagine something that does not exist.

The mind can create and fantasize a mental reality that is an illusion. Problems can arise if these "castles in the air" are used as true reality. In the yoga literature one often uses an example with a rope taken for a snake to illustrate this. In the dark one is mistaken thinking that a rope is a snake which evokes fear. When the light is turned on, you see reality, ie. that the thing on the floor is a rope and that the snake is a mental illusion.

10. Sleep (nidrā) is the mental state characterized by the absence of awareness.

The dreamless sleep is characterized by non-mental activity.

अनुभूतविषयासम्प्रमोषः स्मृतिः॥११॥

11. Anubhūta-viṣayāsampramoṣaḥ smṛtiḥ

अभ्यासवैराग्याभ्यां तन्निरोधः॥१२॥

12. Abhyāsa-vairāgyābhyāṁ tan-nirodhaḥ

तत्र स्थितौ यत्नोऽभ्यासः॥१३॥

13. Tatra sthitau yatno'bhyāsaḥ

स तु दीर्घकालनैरन्तर्यसत्कारासेवितो दृढभूमिः॥१४॥

14. Sa tu dīrgha-kāla-nairantarya-satkārāsevito
drdha-bhūmiḥ

दृष्टानुश्रवकविषियवतृष्णस्य वशीकारसञ्ज्ञा
वैराग्यम्॥१५॥

15. Dṛṣṭānuśravika-viṣaya-vitṛṣṇasya vaśīkāra-
sañjñā vairāgyam

11. Memory (smrti) is the mental ability to become aware of past experiences.

Memory is a tool for the intellect that needs memory to be able to draw conclusions from previous experiences.

12. These sensory sensations can be mastered through practice and attitude.

To be bound to the mind means to be a victim in the relative existence. This does not mean that the mind will be destroyed. The mind with its senses is an excellent tool for navigating in the relative existence. Witnessing the mind by being consciously present in the Consciousness means that one can master the mind. Practicing this approach leads to liberation.

13. By practicing and exercising (abhyāsa) conditions for presence in consciousness arise.

Becoming aware of Consciousness can happen in different ways. One way to become aware is to practice different exercises.

14. Practicing regularly and with dedication for a long time, provides a solid foundation.

Practicing can mean being vigilant and present. It enables an awareness, which provides a stable foundation. The reason for vigilance is that the mind and senses constantly want all the attention, which can mean that the awareness of Consciousness is lost.

15. When independence (vairāgyā) prevails, awareness is no longer bound by the senses and can then be present in Consciousness. This is a state of self-sufficiency. There is then no need to seek sensual satisfaction.

When awareness can be present in Consciousness, freedom and self-sufficiency arise. There is then no need to search for pleasures, wealth and power. In this state of Consciousness, it is obvious that pleasures, possessions and positions of power do not provide real freedom and satisfaction.

तत्परं पुरुषख्यातेर्गुणवैतृष्ण्यम् ॥१६॥

16. Tat paraṁ puruṣa-khyāter guṇavaitṛṣṇyam

वितर्कविचारानन्दास्मितारूपानुगमात्सम्प्रज्ञातः ॥१७॥

17. Vitarka-vicārānandāsmitārūpānugamāt
samprajñātaḥ

विरामप्रत्ययाभ्यासपूर्वः संस्कारशेषोऽन्यः ॥१८॥

18. Virāma pratyayābhyāsa-pūrvaḥ
saṁskāra-śeṣo'nyaḥ

भवप्रत्ययो विदेहप्रकृतलियानाम् ॥१९॥

19. Bhavapratyayo videhaprakṛtilayānām

*16. By experiencing Purusa (Consciousness) a state of
freedom arises when the attachment to the qualities of
the relative changing existence (gunas) has ceased.*

*In this state of independence, the mind, ego, intellect
and body continue to function, even they continue to
function in a more harmonious and coordinated way,
but they are no longer an obstacle to the presence of
Consciousness. By experiencing Consciousness, which
is free from all influence and the three gunas, the true
identity is experienced, which witnesses the relative
sensory sensations without being bound by them and
the relatively changing existence, the three gunas. These
qualities and energies are; tamas which is characterized as inertia, cruelty and low energy, rajas as activity,
desire and active energy and sattva as goodness, truth
and pure energy. It is always one of the three gunas that
dominates the present in the relative existence.*

*17. Samprajñātah samādhi, is called the state of Cons-
ciousness that integrates insight and wisdom as well as
happiness with the experience of Consciousness.*

*In this state of Consciousness, which is free from at-
tachment, understanding and insights come as a matter
of course. No intellectual processing is required and
no external information, from e.g. literature or from*

a teacher. Happiness and peace arise spontaneously without any sensation being the cause.

18. In Asamprajñāta-samādhi there are no sensory sensations, but memories of past experiences remain.

The state of Consciousness Samādhi does not mean an extinction of individuality. Experiences and memories that make up the individual's life history and experience bank are still latent.

19. There are those called videhas and prakrtilayas who have innate abilities that enable them to be reconciled with nature without practice and explanation.

For some people, the insight and understanding of the relationship between the observer, the observed and the process of observing is so established and obvious that no explanations or exercises are needed to experience it.

शरद्धावीर्यस्मृतिसिमाधप्रिज्ञापूर्वक इतरेषाम्॥२०॥

20. Śraddhā-vīrya-smṛti-samādhi-prajñāpūrvaka
itareṣām

तीव्रसंवेगानामासन्नः॥२१॥

21. Tīvra-saṁvegānām āsannaḥ

मृदुमध्याधिमात्रत्वात्ततोऽपि विशेषः॥२२॥

22. Mṛdu-madhyādhimātratvāt tato 'pi viśeṣaḥ

ईश्वरप्रणिधानाद्वा॥२३॥

23. Īśvara-praṇidhānād vā

क्लेशकर्मवपिाकाशयैरपरामृष्टः पुरुषविशेष
ईश्वरः॥२४॥

24. Kleśakarmavipākāśayairaparāmṛṣṭaḥ
puruṣaviśeṣa īśvaraḥ

*20. Others use knowledge, trust and spiritual discipline
to establish the Asamprajñāta-samādhi level of consciousness.*

*Being focused and present is the basis for being aware
of the consciousness. Knowledge, trust and spiritual
discipline are tools that can be helpful.*

*21. He who is focused and has a strong desire soon
reaches the state of consciousness samādhi.*

*If the desire is strong and established on an active cons-
cious level, life will be focused on satisfying this desire as
soon as possible.*

*22. The degree of commitment to reach samādhi, varies
from small to moderate or intense.*

*At different times during a life cycle, the conditions can
vary when it comes to focusing on and devoting time to,
a commitment to reach Samādhi. Both the prevailing
life situation and the intensity of the desire to reach
samādhi affect the intensity of the yoga practice.*

*23. By surrendering to Īśvara (the consciousness of
God), realization can also take place.*

When awareness is present in Consciousness, Samādhi is a fact. This association is not bound to anything that will happen in the future as Consciousness is already present and has always existed. It is not something that needs to be created or developed but can be experienced here and now, but there must be a desire and a willingness to cooperate to surrender to God. This is called Bhakti Yoga.

24. Īśvara is not bound by karma and suffering.
Īśvara is a personal aspect of Purusa (Consciousness). But this divine personality is not affected like other personalities by karma. The meaning of karma is that actions create repercussions that affect the individual. Karma is a way of educating the individual through problems and suffering creating desires for a better life situation. Īśvara which is already perfect and self-sufficient does not need to be nurtured through karma.

तत्र निरतिशयं सर्वज्ञत्ववीजम्॥२५॥

25. Tatra niratiśayaṁ sarvajñatva beejam

पूर्वेषामपि गुरुः कालेनानवच्छेदात्॥२६॥

26. Sa pūrveṣāmapi guruḥ kālenānavacchedāt

तस्य वाचकः प्रणवः॥२७॥

27. Tasya vācakaḥ praṇavaḥ

तज्जपस्तदर्थभावनम्॥२८॥

28. Tajjapas tad-artha-bhāvanam

ततः प्रत्यक्चेतनाधिगमोऽप्यन्तरायाभावश्च॥२९॥

29. Tataḥ pratyak-cetanādhigamo'py an-
tarāyā-bhāvaś ca

25. Īśvara, is the seed of the origin of everything, is
omniscient.

The God-consciousness has total knowledge, control and
presence both in the manifested relative existence and
the absolute being, the unmanifested existence.
26. The divine, independent of time, is the teacher of the
teachers of all ages.

The knowledge transmitted from the consciousness of
God is independent of time. It is independent of the
prevailing spirit of the times. This means that the same
knowledge is conveyed from the consciousness of God
regardless of the age that prevails. What may vary is the
susceptibility that may be different in different eras.

27. The divine manifests itself as pranavah in the form
of Āum (Om).

Āum or Om is a sound that has the quality and energy
of the divine and that permeates and vibrates throughout the whole of relative existence. It is a "divine music"
that one can pay attention to and use as a mantra in
meditation.

28. One should constantly repeat and pay attention to
Om.

Focusing and keeping attention on the mantra Om, means that the mantra´s qualities and energy have prescence in the mind. There are then conditions for contact with Consciousness.

29. In this way the obstacles can be removed and then the possibility arises that Consciousness can be experienced.

The effects of being focused and present in Om can be both mental and physical healing. In this way, attention can go from problems and suffering to experiencing Consciousness as the real and true identity.

व्याधिस्त्यानसंशयप्रमादालस्याविरतिभ्रा
न्तिदर्शनालब्धभूमिकत्वानवस्थितत्वानि
चित्तविक्षेपास्तेऽन्तरायाः ॥३०॥

30. Vyādhi- styāna-saṁśaya-pramādālasyā-vira-
ti-bhrānti-darśanālabdhabhūmi-katvānavasthitat-
vāni citta-vikṣepās te 'ntarāyāḥ

दुःखदौर्मनस्याङ्गमेजयत्वश्वासप्रश्वासा
विक्षेपसहभुवः ॥३१॥

31. Duḥkha-daurmanasyāṅgamejayatva-śvāsa-
praśvāsā vikṣepa-sahabhuvaḥ

तत्प्रतिषिधार्थमेकतत्त्वाभ्यासः ॥३२॥

32. Tat-pratiṣedhārtham eka-tattvābhyāsaḥ

मैत्रीकरुणामुदितोपेक्षाणां
सुखदुःखपुण्यापुण्यविषयाणां
भावनातश्चित्तप्रसादनम् ॥३३॥

33. Maitrī-karuṇā-muditopekṣāṇāṁ sukha-duḥk-
ha-puṇyāpuṇya-viṣayāṇāṁ bhāvanātaś-cit-
ta-prasādanam

30. *Illness, lethargy, doubt, thoughtlessness, listlessness, delusion, difficulty in concentrating and instability are the factors that appear to be obstacles.*

The nine factors listed are characteristics of a awareness that is bound to the mind and lacks conscious anchoring in Consciousness. Since these factors are obstacles, they must be a way out of this mental prison.

31. *Suffering, anxiety, tremors in the body and irregular breathing may be the result of this state of Consciousness.*

This state of Consciousness eventually results in an overload in the nervous system, which then causes problems in various bodily functions and mental disorders. Today we usually call this condition "stress".

32. *Removing these obstacles requires focused and regular practice.*

Getting out of that mental prison may require a regular commitment of being focused and present in appropriate exercises, in order to thereby make the awareness change focus.

33. *When peace and quiet prevail, the reaction to the*

surroundings takes on these qualities; kindness and fellowship with the happy, compassion and love for the unhappy and suffering, neutrality and indifference to the wicked.

Evil can be dealt with in different ways; meeting evil with evil reinforces evil, meeting it with love can in some cases reduce evil, but in other situations evil can be strengthened by feeling threatened. Approaching evil with neutrality and indifference can mean that evil remains latent and inactive. To behave consciously present rooted in the Consciousness, adapted to the prevailing situation, is the best approach, to evil.

परच्छर्दनवधिारणाभ्यां वा प्राणस्य॥३४॥

34. Pracchardana-vidhāraṇābhyāṁ vā prāṇasya

विषियवती वा प्रवृत्तिरुत्पन्ना मनसः
स्थतिनिबिन्धनी॥३५॥

35.Viṣayavatī vā pravṛttir utpannā manasaḥ st-
hiti-nibandhainī

वशोका वा ज्योतष्मिती॥३६॥

36. Viśokā vā jyotiṣmatī

वीतरागवषियं वा चत्तिम्॥३७॥

37. Vīta-rāga-viṣayaṁ vā cittam

स्वप्ननदिराज्ञानालम्बनं वा॥३८॥

38. Svapna-nidrā-jñānālambanaṁ vā

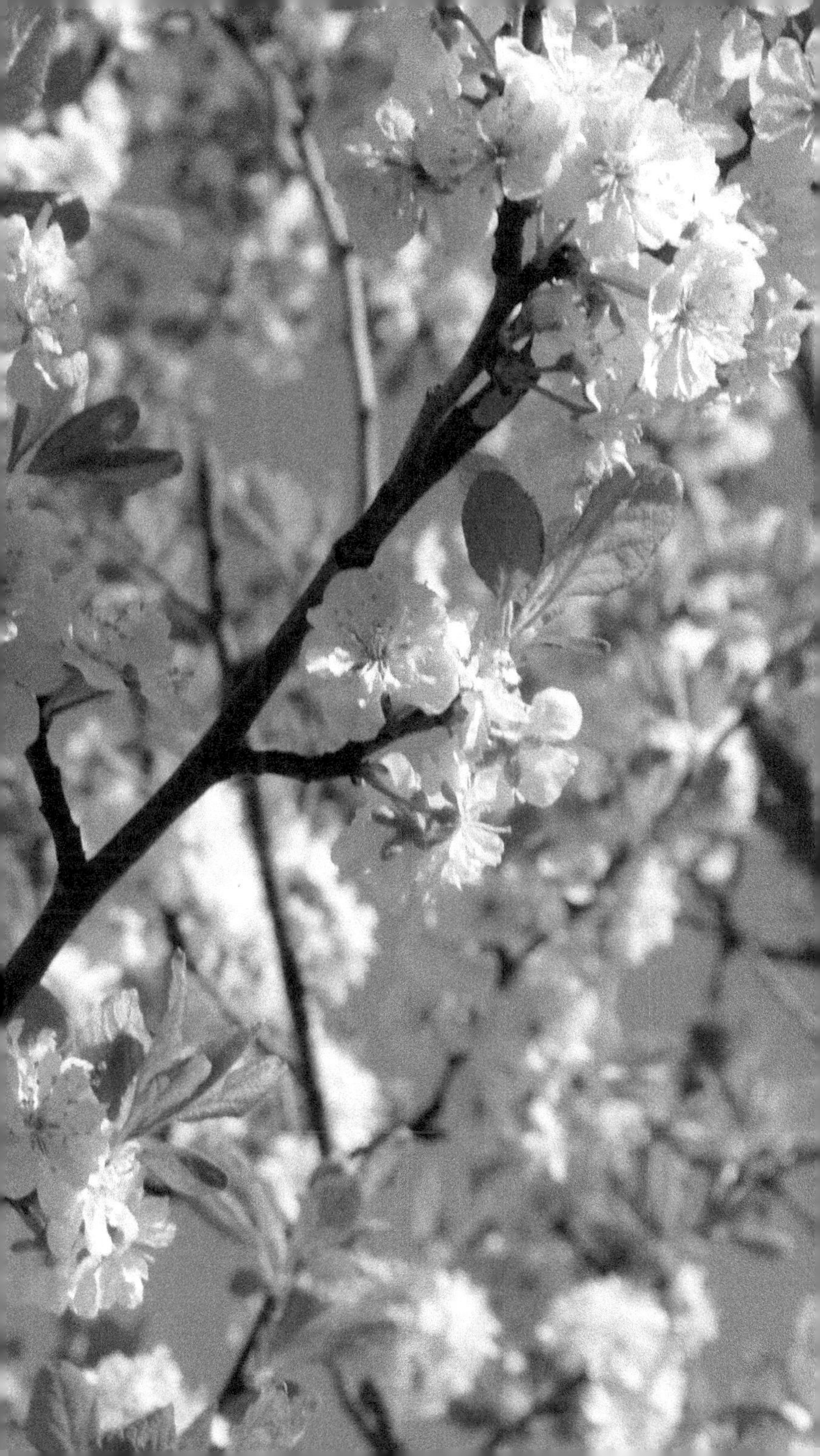

34. Peace and quiet can be obtained by focusing on breathing.

Applying breathing exercises (pranayama) is an effective method of taking attention from sensory sensations to presence in the mind, which results in peace and quiet.

35. When awareness is present at more subtle levels of Consciousness, silence and stability are established.

As awareness begins to come into contact with consciousness, a characteristic is that sensory activity decreases and an inner stillness arises. This stillness is not dependent on external circumstances. The flow of thoughts decreases and thoughts come only when they fill a necessary need.

36. When awareness is not bound by sorrow and suffering, inner light can be experienced.

An inner enlightenment can be experienced in certain states of consciousness. It is not an external physical light that is conveyed via the visual sense, but an inner light that can be experienced as concretely as external light impulses.

37. Paying attention to someone who is free from

attachment and desire can lead to awareness becoming focused and present.

Paying attention to someone who is free from attachment and desire can be a help to be able to experience the level of consciousness where there is freedom from attachment and desire. Meeting such a person can mean that this happens spontaneously, but it can also happen at a distance through the invocation in prayer or during meditation. Even reading a text that such a person has written or reading stories about the person in question can affect. Looking at the person in a picture or film can also have such an effect. Therefore, people have always experienced an attraction to saints.

38. If Consciousness is present during sleep or dreamless sleep, this will allow new insights and knowledge and thus stability can be established.

During dream and dreamless sleep, the five senses are not active and thus do not take attention. Thus, awareness can have the opportunity to share knowledge from Consciousness that can provide new insights and contribute to presence in Consciousness. That contributes to stability.

यथाभिमतध्यानाद्वा॥३९॥

39. Yathābhimata-dhyānād vā

परमाणुपरममहत्त्वान्तोऽस्य वशीकारः॥४०॥

40. Paramāṇu-parama-mahattvānto'sya vaśīkāraḥ

क्षीणवृत्तेरभिजातस्येव मणेर्ग्रहीतृग्रहणग्राह्येषु
तत्स्थतदञ्जनता समापत्तिः॥४१॥

41. Kṣīṇa-vṛtter abhijātasyeva maṇer grahītṛ-gra-
haṇa-grāhyeṣu tatstha-tadañjanatā samāpattiḥ

शब्दार्थज्ञानविकल्पैः सङ्कीर्णा सवितर्का
समापत्तिः॥४२॥

42. Tatra śabdārtha-jñāna-vikalpaiḥ saṅkīrṇā savitarkā samāpattiḥ

*39. Also by paying attention to some dear object this
state of consciousness can be achieved.*

*There are many different meditationtechniques that can
be applied to keep focused and present. It can be on an
object, e.g. on a picture of a saint, a flame of fire, on the
function of breathing and exhalation or mentally, on a
sound or a word (a mantra).*

*40. The ability to be consciously present in Conscio-
usness provides the possibility of being present in the
smallest atom up to the infinitely large universe.
When awareness is present in Consciousness there are
no limitations. Then time and space do not constitute
mental limitations.*

*41. Consciousness is like a crystal which is in itself
transparent but which reflects colors from the surroundings. When the senses have ceased to color and bind
the consciousness, the ability to distinguish between the
observer, the ability to observe and the observed arises.*

*When awareness is established in Consciousness the
state of consciousness is no longer colored and bound
by relative existence. Being independent and unaffected
by the relative existence, enables the consciousness to
be able to meet sensory sensations by distinguishing*

between the observer, the ability to observe and the observed. Of course, senses and mental activity continue to act, but a conscious presence is now established that observes this activity.

42. Savitarkā samāpattihis the state of consciousness in which there is a confusion of the true meaning of a word, its assumed meaning, and its quality.

In the state of consciousness called savitarkā samāpattih there is uncertainty about the true meaning of a word. In this state the knowledge of the word is not rooted in a level of pure Consciousness that is linked to consciousness.

समृतपरिशुद्धौ स्वरूपशून्येवार्थमात्रनिर्भासा
निर्वितर्का॥४३॥

43. Smṛti-pariśuddhau svarūpa-śūny-
evārtha-mātra-nirbhāsā nirvitarkā

एतयैव सविचारा निर्विचारा च सूक्ष्मवषिया
व्याख्याता॥४४॥

44. Etayaiva savicārā nirvicārā ca sūkṣmaviṣayā
vyākhyātā

सूक्ष्मवषियत्वं चालङ्गिपर्यवसानम्॥४५॥

45. Sūkṣma-viṣayatvaṁ cāliṅga-pary-avasānam

ता एव सवीजः समाधिः॥४६॥

46. Tā eva savījaḥ samādhiḥ

निर्विचारवैशारद्येऽध्यात्मपरसादः॥४७॥

47. Nirvicāra-vaiśāradye 'dhyātma-prasādaḥ

*43. Nirvitarka Samadhi is called the state of conscio-
usness which enables true knowledge of an object to be
experienced by the memory being pure and clear and
the attention present without anything distracting it.*

*When awareness is rooted in Consciousness an object
can be experienced as it is without having it to be jud-
ged through the mind and previous experiences.*

*44. Savicāra and nirvicāra samadhi are states of consci-
ousness that arise when attention is focused on a subtle
object.*

*The fact that an object is subtle may mean that it cannot
be experienced by the sense organs or that it cannot be
understood by the intellect. Its existence is beyond the
perceptual capacity of the mind, but can be experienced
on a more subtle level of consciousness.*

*45. Beyond the experience of the objects' most subtle
state in the manifested nature (prakriti), there is alinga
(the unmanifest).*

*The relative manifested existence is governed by nature
(prakriti) which is encompassed by (gunas) the three different energies tamas, rajas and sattva. Beyond prakriti
there are alinga ie. the unmanifest.*

*46. These levels of Consciousness (samādhis) can be seen
as basic 'seeds'.*

*These mentioned levels of Consciousness (samādhis) can
be seen as a seed but it has not yet resulted in a fully
developed established plant. Awareness is not yet firmly
anchored and present in Consciousness.*

*47. In the state of consciousness called nirvicāra a
purification occurs which enables contact with Consciousness.*

*Through conscious presence and focusing on more subtle
levels of consciousness, a purification process begins that
result in the removal of stress and tension, both physically and mentally. As a result, the conditions for contact
with Consciousness increase.*

ऋतम्भरा तत्र प्रज्ञा॥४८॥

48. Ṛtambharā tatra prajñā

श्रुतानुमानप्रज्ञाभ्यामन्यवषिया
वशिेषार्थत्वात्॥४९॥

49. Śrutānumāna-prajñābhyām anya-viṣayā
viśeṣārthatvāt

तज्जः संस्कारोऽन्यसंस्कारप्रतिबिन्धी॥५०॥

50. Tajjaḥ saṁskāro 'nya-saṁskāra-pratibandhī

तस्यापि निरोधे सर्वनिरोधान्निर्वीजः समाधिः॥५१॥

51. Tasyāpi nirodhe sarva-nirodhān nirvījaḥ samādhiḥ

48. At this level of consciousness, rtambharā prajñā is experienced, which means truth and knowledge.
The truth and knowledge of Consciousness is not relative and not linked to the intellectual conditions of the mind to acquire knowledge and truth. The wisdom of Consciousness is experienced as an obvious insight that comes when one is mature enough to receive it.

49. The knowledge obtained through the level of consciousness in rtambharā does not depend on intellectual inference but comes directly from Consciousness. Intellectual guidance and knowledge from teachers as well as books convey knowledge that is of course also needed in the relative existence, but knowledge and insights that convey spiritual clarity and understanding come directly from Consciousness.

50. When awareness is present in the state of consciousness ritambharā, all sensory impressions are dissipated.

When awareness and Consciousness are united, this state overshadows all other states of consciousness. Sensory sensations and latent senses are then no longer dominant.

51. Once this awareness of Consciousness is established, there is no longer any "seed" to develop. This samādhi means liberation from birth and death.

When awareness of Consciousness is completed and established, there is nothing more to realize. The school of life has ended teaching and then no more lessons are needed and thus no more incarnations in the relative existence. Awareness no longer experiences any dualism in relation to Consciousness.

Chapter 2

SADHANA PADA

To practice yoga exercises

तपःस्वाध्यायेश्वरप्ररणधिानानि क्रियायोगः॥१॥

1. Tapaḥ-svādhyāyeśvara-praṇidhānāni
kriyā-yogaḥ

समाधभिावनार्थः क्लेशतनूकरणार्थश्च॥२॥

2. Samādhi bhāvanārthaḥ kleśa-tanūkara-ṇārthaś
ca

अवद्यिास्मतिारागद्वेषाभनिविशाः पञ्च क्लेशाः॥३॥

3. Avidyā asmitā-rāga-dveṣābhiniveśāḥ pañca
kleśāḥ

अवद्यिा क्षेत्रमुत्तरेषां प्रसुप्ततनुवच्छिन्निनोदाराणा
म्॥४॥

4. Avidyā kṣetram uttareṣāṁ prasupta-tanu-vic-
chinnodārāṇām

अनत्यिाशुचदिुःखानात्मसु नत्यिशुचसिुखात्मख्यातरि
वद्यिा॥५॥

5. Anityāśuci duḥkhānātmasu nitya-śuci-sukhātma
khyātir avidyā

*1. Self-discipline, study and surrender to Īśvara (God)
enables yoga.*

*To be focused and ambitious in the practice of spiritual,
purifying exercises, and to study holy scriptures, and to
surrender to the consciousness of God, is to focus attention on yoga. These are paths for union and identification with Consciousness.*

*2. This practition brings attention to Samādhi and it
minimizes suffering.*

*As long as states of awareness have the desire for
pleasures and sensory objects are dominant and satisfy,
life will consist of suffering. The medicine against this is
rooted in the Samadhi state of Consciousness.*

*3. Kleśāh(suffering) is due to avidyā (ignorance) and
results in asmitā (egoism), rāga (bondage), dvesa (aversion) and abhiniveśah(death anxiety).*

*As long as awareness is bound to the mind, avidyā
prevails, ie. There is ignorance of identity with Consciousness. In this state of awareness, the ego dominates. As
the will and desires of the ego do not always correspond
to the reality of the present, conflict and suffering arise.
The will and desires of the ego also come into conflict*

with an imagined future. Because the ego sees its exis-tence limited to time and space, death is the worst that can occur, which causes death anxiety as it means the end of the ego.

4. Avidyā (ignorance) is the cause of suffering which can be dormant, diminishing or active and increasing.

When consciousness is rooted in the mind, the life situa-tion shifts between happiness and joy as well as suffe-ring. As there are periods of happiness and joy, suffering still remains latent.

5. Ignorance is to identify with non-ātma (non-self) instead of ātma (Self) and to confuse the temporary with the eternal, the unclean with the pure, and suffe-ring as enjoyable.

The state of ignorance is characterized by mental confusion and is an illusory state. To be identified with non-ātma (non-self) instead of ātma (Self) means to be anchored in the mind instead of Consciousness.

दृग्दर्शनशक्त्योरेकात्मतेवास्मिता॥६॥

6. Dṛg-darśana-śaktyor ekātmatevāsmitā

सुखानुशयी रागः॥७॥

7. Sukhānuśayī rāgaḥ

दुःखानुशयी द्वेषः॥८॥

8. Duḥkhānuśayī dveṣaḥ

स्वरसवाही विदुषोऽपि तथारूढोऽभिनिवेशः॥९॥

9. Svarasavāhī viduṣo 'pi tathā rūḍho 'bhiniveśaḥ

ते प्रतिप्रसवहेयाः सूक्ष्माः॥१०॥

10. Te pratiprasava-heyāḥ sūkṣmāḥ

6. *Asmitā (individuality, egoism) arises when the mind
and intellect, thinks itself to be ātma (the Self or Consciousness), this confusion then becomes an obstacle to the
experience of Consciousness.*

*When awareness is rooted in an identity that has been
created by the mind, intellect and ego, this identity
becomes relative and limited. Individuality arises
through the assumption that this relative and limited
state of awareness is the real self. The real self is in fact
not relative and limited but absolute and eternally pure
Consciousness.*

7. *Bondage arises through desire.*

*Some desires can bind awareness to the mind and beco-
me an obstacle to the experience of Consciousness.*

8. *Out of suffering arises aversion.*

*An ongoing suffering often creates a negative mood and
low energy.*

9. *Death anxiety and the need to cling to life are present
in all of us, even in the wise.*

Anxiety about death and the will to live are strongly

established in every human being. If breathing ceases, there will automatically be death anxiety to protect life.

10. These obstacles disappear when awareness is rooted in Consciousness.

Suffering and ignorance exist as long as awareness is rooted in the mind. To be present in Consciousness means to no longer be bound by suffering and ignorance.

ध्यानहेयास्तद्वृत्तयः॥११॥

11. Dhyāna-heyās-tad-vṛttayaḥ

क्लेशमूलः कर्माशयो दृष्टादृष्टजन्मवेदनीयः॥१२॥

12. Kleśa-mūlaḥ karmāśayo dṛṣṭādṛṣṭa-janmave-
danīyaḥ

सति मूले तद्विपाको जात्यायुर्भोगाः॥१३॥

13. Sati mūle tad-vipāko jāty-āyur-bhogāḥ

ते ह्लादपरितापफलाः पुण्यापुण्यहेतुत्वात्॥१४॥

14. Te hlāda-paritāpa-phalāḥ puṇyāpuṇya-hetutvāt

परिणामतापसंस्कारदुःखैर्गुणवृत्तविरोधाच्च दुःखमेव
सर्वं विविकनिः॥१५॥

15. Pariṇāma-tāpa-saṁskāra-duḥkhair guṇa-vṛt-
ti-virodhāc ca duḥkham eva sarvaṁ vivekinaḥ

*11. To anchor awareness in Consciousness to get rid of
anxiety and suffering can be done through meditation.*

*Allowing attention to be present in Consciousness
through meditation can be a way to get rid of anxiety
and stress that causes suffering.*

*12. Karmāśaya (karma) are experiences that are latent
and expressed in action in this life or in future life.*

*What has been done cannot be undone, therefore life
cannot be in any other way than it is right now. The law
of karma is relentless and cannot be negotiated away.
Sooner or later comes the effect of an act. This applies
to both an individual and to a collective level. At the
level of the mind, one may think that "no one knows" or
"one has soon forgotten". But everything that happens is
registered and not forgotten, by the observer at the level
of Consciousness.*

*13. As long as there is stored karma, this karma will
manifest itself in the form of birth and a life cycle of
actions.*

*The stored quota of karma (the bank of experience)
wants to manifest itself in a life situation and therefore
there is a reason for birth. All desires that have not been*

allowed to manifest themselves are waiting for an opportunity to become established.

14. Good or bad karma results in happiness and suffering respectively.

Karma is like seeds that are sown in soil and begin to germinate into a plant. The plant can become a thorny shrub or a beautiful flower depending on the conditions of the seed.

15. He who observes sees that all relative experiences lead to suffering and anxiety no matter which of the three gunas dominates, and that enjoyable moods are transient.

हेयं दुःखमनागतम्॥१६॥

16. Heyaṁ duḥkha manāgatam

दरष्टृदृश्ययोः संयोगो हेयहेतुः॥१७॥

17. Draṣṭr̥-dr̥śyayoḥ saṁyogo heya-hetuḥ

प्रकाशक्रयिास्थतिशीलं भूतेन्द्रयिात्मकं
भोगापवर्गार्थं दृश्यम्॥१८॥

18. Prakāśa-kriyā-sthiti-śīlaṁ bhūtendriyāt-makaṁ
bhogāpavargārthaṁ dr̥śyam

वशिषावशिषलङ्गिमात्रालङ्गिानि गुणपर्वाणि॥१९॥

19. Viśeṣāviśeṣa-liṅgamātrāliṅgāni guṇa-parvāṇi

दरष्टा दृशमिात्रः शुद्धोऽपि प्रत्ययानुपश्यः॥२०॥

20. Draṣṭā dr̥śimātraḥ śuddho 'pi pratyayā-nu-
paśyaḥ

*16. Suffering that has not yet manifested can be avoided.
Being rooted in the mind means that both good and
bad karma affect the presence in the present. Karma
manifests itself as impulses that want to become aware
and manifested. He who is rooted in Consciousness has
the opportunity to be unaffected by these impulses and
can therefore avoid the consequences of karma.
17. The cause of suffering is that the observer identifies
with what is observed.*

*As long as the observer identifies with the observation,
ie. with the mind and with the senses, there is duality
and thus a prerequisite for suffering. When the observer
is rooted in Consciousness, there is no longer any duality
and thus there is no conflict that can create suffering.*

*18. What can be observed is the relative existence of the
five elements and the energies of tamas, rajas and sat-
vas. The purpose of its existence is to provide experiences that lead to liberation.*

*The purpose of experiences that lead to liberation is to
be liberated from being enslaved by the mind and its
desires, in order to be present in the absolute eternal
existence of Consciousness.*

19. The three gunas affect awareness with impulses or

*sensations that can be subtle or gross, perceptible or
unconscious.*

*Some impulses from the three gunas can be understood
intellectually and can be put into words, while others are
perceived on a subtle emotional level.*

*20. Pure Consciousness is untouched as it witnesses the
mind and the senses.*

*When awareness is anchored in Consciousness what is
happening in the present is witnessed and then freedom
arises to decide whether the sensory sensations are to
be manifested or not. This means that the mind cannot
enslave Consciousness. Only then does real freedom and
understanding arise such as; that the mind no longer
alone affects the event.*

तदर्थ एव दृश्यस्यात्मा॥२१॥

21. Tad-artha eva dṛśyasyātmā

कृतार्थं प्रति नष्टमप्यनष्टं
तदन्यसाधारणत्वात्॥२२॥

22. Kṛtārthaṁ prati naṣṭam apy anaṣṭaṁ
tad-anya-sādhāraṇatvāt

स्वस्वामिशक्त्योः स्वरूपोपलब्धिहेतुः संयोगः॥२३॥

23. Sva-svāmi-śaktyoḥ svarūpopalabdhi-hetuḥ
saṁyogaḥ

तस्य हेतुरविद्या॥२४॥

24. Tasya hetur avidyā

तदभावात्संयोगाभावो हानं तद्दृशेः कैवल्यम्॥२५॥

25. Tad-abhāvāt saṁyogābhāvo hānaṁ tad dṛśeḥ
kaivalyam

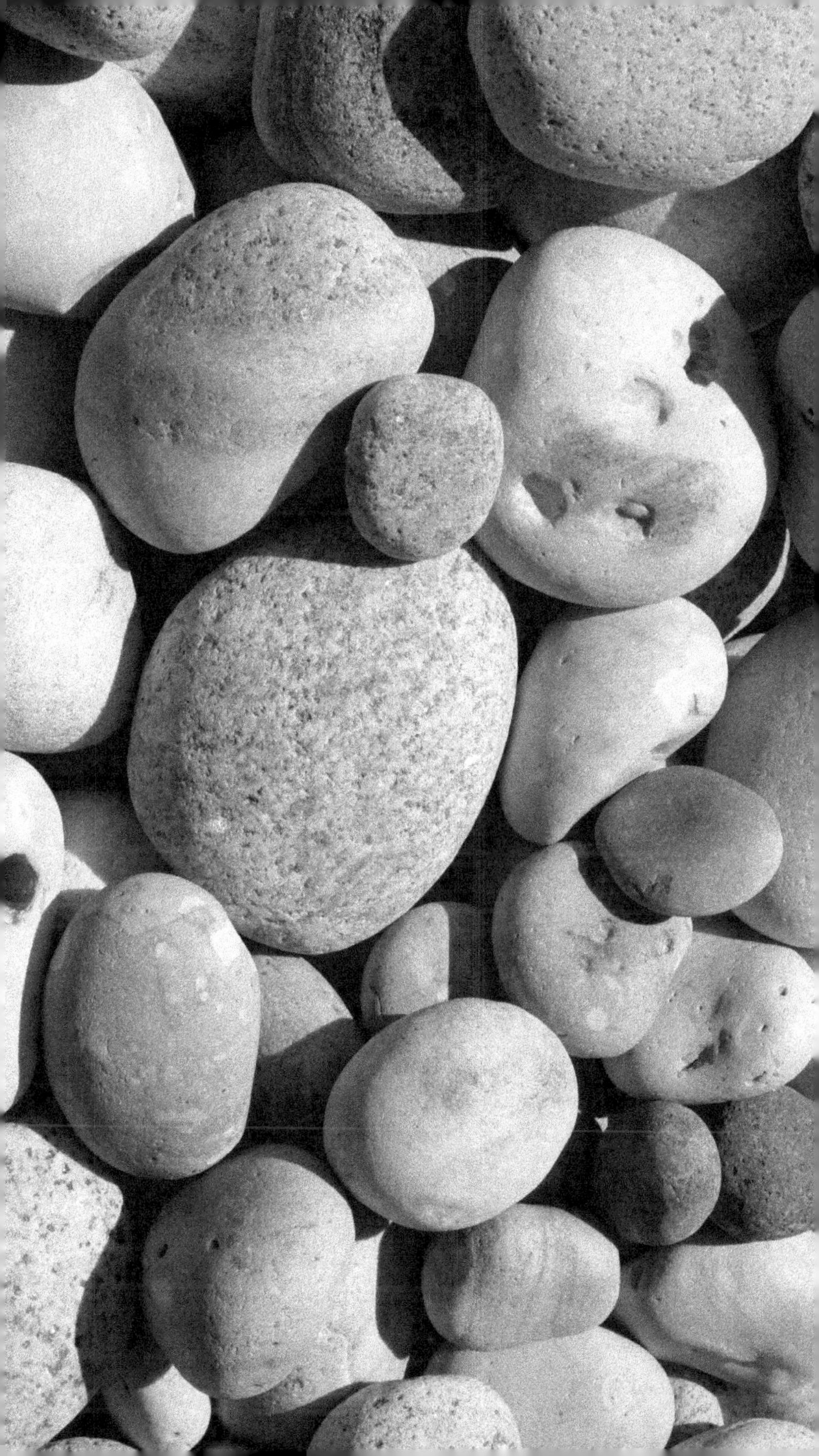

21. *The manifested exists for Consciousness (ātmān).*

The world and relative existence exist as mental sensory sensations for consciousness.

22. *The mental sensations are not real to the one who is present in the Consciousness, while they are reality to the one who is bound to the mind.*

Life is experienced differently depending on the level of awareness on which the experience is based.

23. *When the observer observes what is observed, the true identity of both the observer and the observed is experienced.*

When awareness is present in Consciousness, ie. the observer, the true identity of both the observer and the observed is revealed.

24. *Identifying with what is observed depends on ignorance.*

As long as one identifies with body and mind, reality is obscured by ignorance. It is not an intellectual ignorance but an experiential ignorance, ie. it is about lack of experience in identifying with the observer. .

25. *When the identification with the observer becomes conscious, the ignorance disappears and the awareness is liberated and enlightened.*

विविकख्यातिरिवप्लिवा हानोपायः॥२६॥

26. Viveka-khyātir aviplavā hānopāyaḥ

तस्य सप्तधा प्रान्तभूमिः प्रज्ञा॥२७॥

27. Tasya saptadhā prānta-bhūmiḥ prajñā

योगाङ्गानुष्ठानादशुद्धक्षिये
ज्ञानदीप्तिरिवविकख्यातेः॥२८॥

28. Yogāṅgānuṣṭhānād aśuddhi-kṣaye jñāna-dīptir
ā viveka-khyāteḥ

यमनियमासनप्राणायामप्रत्याहारधारणाध्यानसमाधयोऽष्टावङ्गानि॥

29. Yama-niyamāsana-prāṇāyāma-pra-
tyāhāra-dhāraṇā-dhyāna-samādhayo'ṣṭāv aṅgāni

26. Being constantly anchored in Consciousness enables the ignorance to disappear.

To be constantly aware of Consciousness means that every illusions and that all ignorance do not have the opportunity to affect consciousness.

27. Seven ways can be applied to become aware of Consciousness.

The seven paths can be applied either individually or they can be combined.

28. By practicing these exercises, impurities can be removed and this increases the possibility of being able to be aware of Consciousness and thus have access to the ability to distinguish the real from the unreal.

Practicing these exercises does not automatically guarantee that the awareness can be aware of Consciousness, but the conditions will be better.

29. The eight limbs of yoga are;

yama - properties that provide purity and harmony
niyama - rules of life that provide purity and harmony
āsana - postures

prānāyāma - breathing exercises

*pratyāhāra - to divert attention from the objects of the
mind*

dhāranā - conscious presence beyond the mind

dhyāna - meditation

samādhi - conscious presence in Consciousness

*These eight limbs constitute the eightfold path "ashtanga
yoga".*

अहसिासत्यास्तेयब्रह्मचर्यापरिग्रहा यमाः॥३०॥

30. Ahiṁsā satyāsteya-brahmacaryāparigrahā
yamāḥ

जातिदेशकालसमयानवच्छिन्नाः सार्वभौमा
महाव्रतम्॥३१॥

31. Jāti-deśa-kāla-samayānavacchinnāḥ sār-
vabhaumā mahā-vratam

शौचसन्तोषतपःस्वाध्यायेश्वरप्रणिधानानि
नियमाः॥३२॥

32. Śauca-santoṣa-tapaḥ-svādhyāyeśvara-praṇid-
hānāni niyamāḥ

30. *Yama - qualities that provide inner purity, peace and harmony.*

ahimsā - non-violence
satya - to stick to the truth
asteya - absence of greed
brahmacarya - abstinence (celibacy)
aparigrahāh - not to have a desire to own

Being aware of, and living by, these qualities or rules lays the foundation for a life of peace and harmony.

31. *These yamas are universal laws that are not limited by time, place, environment, or the prevailing situation. Yamas are laws rooted in universal wisdom.*

32. *Niyama - the five rules of life.*

śauca - purity
santosa - contentment
tapas - self-discipline
svādhyāya - self-study
īśvarapranidhānā - surrender to God

Niyama's rules of life are there to facilitate a conscious presence in the Consciousness. To keep body and soul pure through exercise, self-discipline and healthy food,

*to be content with what is and to read scriptures that
contain wisdom, this provides the best conditions for
being able to surrender to God.*

67

वितिर्कबाधने प्रतिपिक्षभावनम् ॥ ३३ ॥

33. Vitarka-bādhane pratipakṣa-bhāvanam

वितिर्का हिंसादयः कृतकारितानुमोदिता
लोभक्रोधमोहपूर्वका मृदुमध्याधमात्रा
दुःखाज्ञानानन्तफला इति प्रतिपिक्षभावनम् ॥ ३४ ॥

34. Vitarkā hiṁsādayaḥ kṛta-kāritānumoditā
lobha-krodha-moha-pūrvakā mṛdu-madhyād-
himātrā duḥkhājñānānanta-phalā iti pratipakṣa-bhāvanam

अहिंसाप्रतिष्ठायां तत्सन्निधौ वैरत्यागः ॥ ३५ ॥

35, Ahiṁsā-pratiṣṭhāyāṁ tat-sannidhau vai-
ra-tyāgaḥ

सत्यप्रतिष्ठायां क्रियाफलाश्रयत्वम् ॥ ३६ ॥

36. Satya-pratiṣṭhāyāṁ kriyā-phalāśrayatvam

अस्तेयप्रतिष्ठायां सर्वरत्नोपस्थानम् ॥ ३७ ॥

37. Asteya-pratiṣṭhāyāṁ sarva-ratnopasthānam

33. When awareness is rooted in negative and bad thoughts these can be neutralized if opposite thoughts become conscious instead.

Negative and bad thoughts are generated through the dysfunctional ego. By being rooted in Consciousness these thoughts can not exist and thoughts based on wisdom become conscious instead.

34. Negative and bad thoughts, feelings, and actions, whether caused by greed, anger, or confusion, can be minor, moderate, or intense. They always lead to suffering and ignorance and therefore it is necessary to pay attention to the opposite.

Paying attention to the opposite means paying attention to Consciousness, whish is not limited by the ego.

35. As awareness is rooted in non-violence (ahimsā), the environment will also cease to be hostile.

The energy that a person present in Consciousness radiates affects everyone in the environment more strongly than the energy that emanates from the one who is rooted in the mind.

36. Being rooted in truth (satya) gives the best result and the fruit of action arises without effort.

He who is established in Consciousness becomes a tool for Consciousness and there is then no other alternative to satya, ie. truth. Action is then no longer an action that has a selfish motive, the action is motivated for the good of the whole. The action is performed without resistance and struggle and is therefore perceived as effortless.

37. Being honest and refraining from stealing (asteya), enables all the wealth needed to arise.

He who is honest creates karma, which means that he gets access to what is needed in the current life situation.

ब्रह्मचर्यप्रतिष्ठायां वीर्यलाभः ॥३८॥

38. Brahmacarya-pratiṣṭhāyāṁ vīrya-lābhaḥ

अपरिग्रहस्थैर्ये जन्मकथन्तासम्बोधः ॥३९॥

39. Aparigraha-sthairye janma-kathantā-sambod-
haḥ

शौचात्स्वाङ्गजुगुप्सा परैरसंसर्गः ॥४०॥

40. Śaucāt svāṅga-jugupsā parair asaṁsargaḥ

सत्त्वशुद्धसौमनस्यैकाग्र्येन्द्रियजयात्मदर्शनयोग्
यत्वानि च ॥४१॥

41. Sattvaśuddhi-saumanasyaikāgryendriya-jayāt-
ma-darśana-yogyatvāni ca

सन्तोषादनुत्तमसुखलाभः ॥४२॥

42. Santoṣādanuttamasukhalābhaḥ

38. *Being established in sexual abstinence (brahmaca-rya) provides spiritual energy.*

The desire for sexual pleasure is a strong energy that takes attention to body and mind. Sexual gratification increases sexual desire. Thus, the awareness of Consciousness can be lost and the spiritual energy that arises when this association is conscious can then also be lost. Being free from sexual desire enables more easyly the presence of Consciousness.

39. *Not having a desire to own (aparigraha) gives knowledge of existence.*

The desire for power and wealth is a strong energy that binds awareness to the mind. This negative energy arises from the mind through the greed of the ego and is the root of many of humanity's problems. Mastering greed provides access to knowledge and wisdom.

40. *When inner purity (śaucā) is achieved, this leads to independence from one's own body and indifference to other bodies.*

As the experience of inner purification dominates awareness one's own body is no longer perceived as something with which one identifies and other bodies are no longer perceived as attractive.

41. Through sattvic purification peace and harmony arise, the ability to be consciously present, control of the mind, and the opportunity to experience Consciousness. The sattvic purification occurs when sattva dominates tamas and rajas. In this pure state are the best spiritual conditions.

42. Satisfaction (santosā) brings the highest happiness. To be established in the pure state, ie. being consciously present in Consciousness gives total contentment and the highest happiness.

कायेन्द्रियसिद्धिरशुद्धिक्षयात्तपसः॥४३॥

43. Kāyendriya-siddhir aśuddhi-kṣayāt tapasaḥ

स्वाध्यायादिष्टदेवतासम्प्रयोगः॥४४॥

44. Svādhyāyād iṣṭa-devatā samprayogaḥ

समाधिसिद्धिरीश्वरप्रणिधानात्॥४५॥

45. Samādhi-siddhir īśvara-praṇidhānāt

स्थिरसुखमासनम्॥४६॥

46. Sthira-sukham āsanam

प्रयत्नशैथिल्यानन्तसमापत्तिभ्याम्॥४७॥

47. Prayatna-śaithilyānanta samāpattibhyām

43. Through spiritual exercises (tapas) impurities are removed and purity is achieved in body and soul. Spiritual exercises can be meditation (yoga dhyana), postures (yoga asana) or breathing exercises (yoga pranayama).

44. Studying spiritual scriptures (svādhyāyā) can lead to union with the divine.

When attention is directed to a scripture that describes the union with the divine Consciousness, a desire may arise to experience this, which can then also result in experience of this union (yoga).

45. The result of devotion to and union with the Divine Consciousness (īśvarapranidhānā) is samādhi.

This level of awareness that results in yoga or samādhi means a state of Consciousness has been achieved that is complete, ie. there is nothing more to look for.

46. The physical position (āsana) should be stable but still comfortable.

By being consciously present in the body, the association with Consciousness is facilitated. Mastering the lotus position (padmāsana) provides a stable and comfortable position that is suitable for meditation.

*47. Through a relaxed attitude awareness of Conscio-
usness can be established and thus eternity can become
conscious.*

*When awareness is no longer present in mental activity
the eternity can become conscious. When the time- and
space-bound mind no longer controls awareness, reality
can manifest itself. Being in a relaxed state of awareness
can be helpful for this process.*

ततो द्वन्द्वानभिघातः॥४८॥
48. Tato dvandvānabhighātaḥ

तस्मिन्सति श्वासप्रश्वासयोर्गतिविच्छेदः
प्राणायामः॥४९॥
49. Tasmin sati śvāsa-praśvāsayor gati-vicchedaḥ
prāṇāyāmaḥ

वाह्याभ्यन्तरस्तम्भवृत्तिः देशकालसङ्ख्याभिः
परिदृष्टो दीर्घसूक्ष्मः॥५०॥
50. Bāhyābhyantara-stambha-vṛttir deśakāla-saṅk-
hyābhiḥ paridṛṣṭo dīrghasūkṣmaḥ

वाह्याभ्यन्तरविषियाक्षेपी चतुरथः॥५१॥
51. Bāhyābhyantara-viṣayākṣepī caturthaḥ

ततः क्षीयते प्रकाशावरणम्॥५२॥
52. Tataḥ kṣīyate prakāśāvaraṇam

48. *When awareness is rooted in Consciousness, the duality of sensory perceptions can be observed and thus they no longer cause bother.*

Being able to observe the duality of sensory perceptions means that it is possible to separate the real from the unreal and thus not become a victim of their delusions.

49. *By practicing breathing exercises (prānāyāma), which involves conscious presence in inhalation and exhalation, the breathing activity is calmed.*

Prānā is the subtle energy that is manifested in the relative existence, ie. life energy. Through breathing exercises, prana can be experienced will then provide harmony and energy.

50. *Breathing (at pranayama) changes depending on time and place and in intensity, it can be experienced as inhalation, exhalation or temporary cessation, it can be experienced as prolonged or short.*

In pranayama, breathing is experienced in three different phases inhalation, exhalation and cessation of breathing, as long as consciousness is present at the level of the respiratory function.

51. The fourth type of pranayama goes beyond the inner and outer spheres.

When this type of pranayama is performed, the conscious presence can leave the level of the respiratory function to the autonomous system, to be aware in Consciousness.

52. In this way, the veil that obscures the inner light can be removed.

The inner light is not a light from any outer object such as the sun or a lamp, but the light from within. This light can be experienced without the visual sense being involved and is experienced as lightning from within.

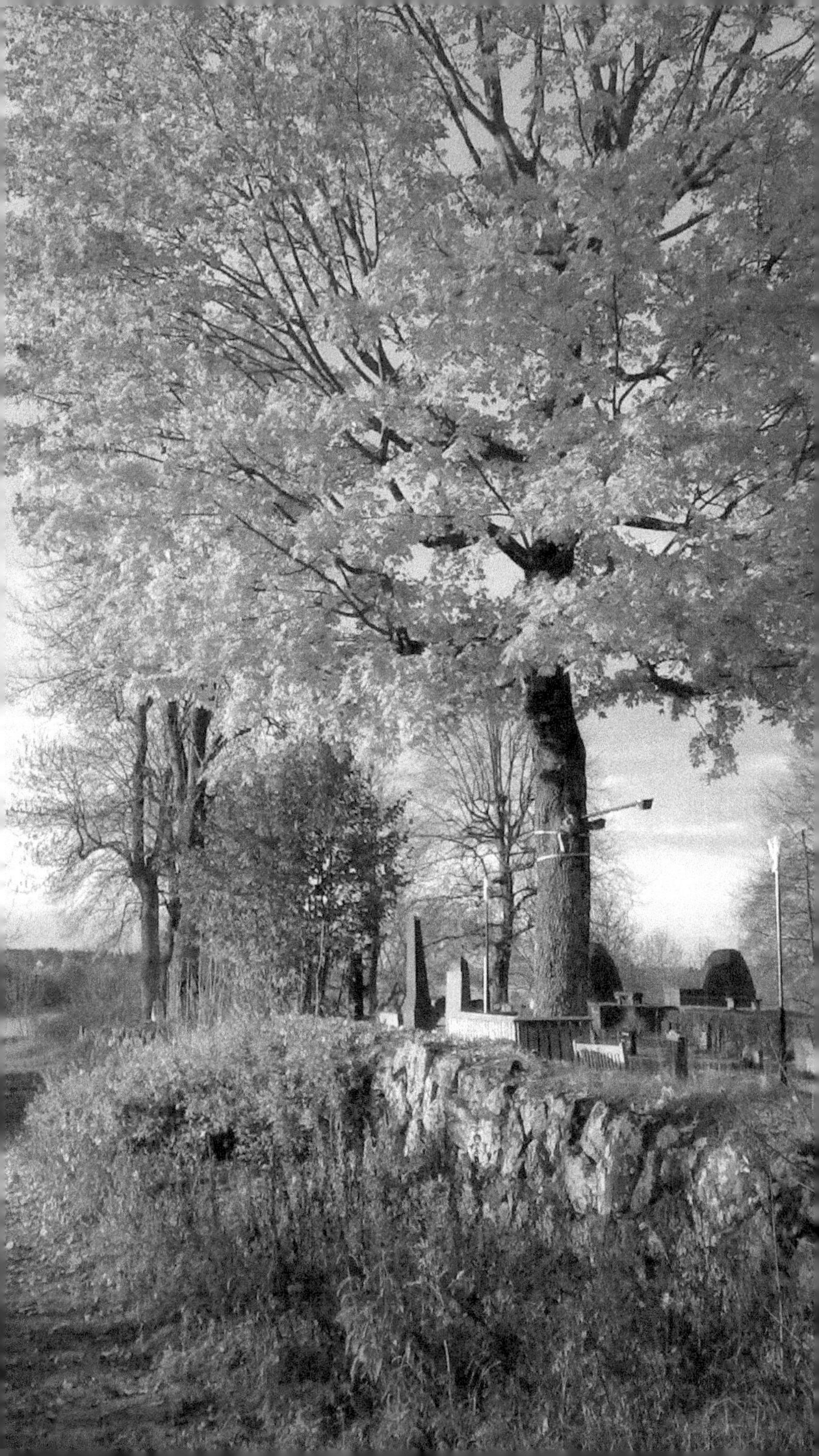

धारणासु च योग्यता मनसः॥५३॥

53. Dhāraṇāsu ca yogyatā manasaḥ

स्वविषयासम्प्रयोगे चित्तस्य स्वरूपानुकार
इवेन्द्रियाणां प्रत्याहारः॥५४॥

54. Sva-viṣayāsamprayoge cittasya sva-
rūpānukāra ivendriyāṇāṁ pratyāhāraḥ

ततः परमा वश्यतेन्द्रियाणाम्॥५५॥

55. Tataḥ paramā vaśyatendriyāṇām

53. Then awareness becomes consciously present
(dhāranā).

This state of consciousness involves presence in the body,
mind and Consciousness.

54. When the senses is drawn away from awareness, this
is called pratyāhāra.

This state of consciousness is characterized by the absence of sensory activity such as thoughts, emotions and
impressions from the sense organs.

55. This state of consciousness involves spontaneous
mastery of the mind.

Trying to control the mind with the help of the intellect
is doomed to fail. By releasing the anchorage in the
intellect and being present in Consciousness, the mind
acquires a subordinate function and then does not
dominate awareness.

Chapter 3

VIBHUTI PADA

Spiritual powers and abilities

देशबन्धश्चत्तितस्य धारणा॥१॥

1. Deśa-bandhaś cittasya dhāraṇā

तत्र प्रत्ययैकतानता ध्यानम्॥२॥

2. Tatra pratyayaikatānatā dhyānam

तदेवार्थमात्रनिर्भासं स्वरूपशून्यमिव समाधिः॥३॥

3. Tad evārthamātra-nirbhāsaṁ svarūpa-śūnyami-
va samādhiḥ

त्रयमेकत्र संयमः॥४॥

4. Trayam ekatra saṁyamaḥ

तज्जयात्प्रज्ञालोकः॥५॥

5. Taj-jayāt prajñālokaḥ

तस्य भूमिषु विनियोगः॥६॥

6. Tasya bhūmiṣu viniyogaḥ

1. To be present is dhāranā.

To concentrate on something is dhāranā.

2. To allow awareness to flow towards a specific object is called meditation (dhyāna).

To be present both in the now and simultaneously let the attention be directed towards the object of meditation means that an association with the object of meditation can take place.

3. When awareness can be reconciled with and is un-disturbed by the meditation object, the state of conscio-usness, samādhi, arises.

If the senses don´t distract when consciousness is united with the object of meditation, awareness of Conscious-ness can arise. This condition is called yoga or samādhi.

4. When these three (dhāranā, dhyāna and samādhi) work together, samyama arises.

Samyama is a condition that can be temporary or permanent.

5. In this state of consciousness there is access to the light of intuitive knowledge.

Intuitive knowledge does not come from e.g. via a book or a teacher but from within and it comes "like lightning from a clear sky". This knowledge does not need to be valued and questioned intellectually.

6. Its (samyama) application takes place via various steps.

Samyama does not arise through intellectual understanding but through practical application and practice.

तरयमन्तरङ्गं पूर्वेभ्यः॥७॥

7. Trayam antarangam pūrvebhyaḥ

तदपि वहिरङ्गं निर्वीजस्य॥८॥

8. Tad api vahir-angam nirvījasya

व्युत्थाननिरोधसंस्कारयोरभिभिवप्रादुर्भावौ
निरोधक्षणचित्तान्वयो निरोधपरिणामः॥९॥

9. Vyutthāna-nirodha-samskāray-
or-abhibha-va-prādurbhāvau nirodha-kṣaṇa-cittān-
vayo nirodha-pariṇāmaḥ

तस्य प्रशान्तवाहिता संस्कारात्॥१०॥

10. Tasya praśānta-vāhitā samskārāt

सर्वार्थतैकाग्रतयोः क्षयोदयौ चित्तस्य
समाधिपरिणामः॥११॥

11. Sarvārthataikāgratayoḥ kṣayodayau cittasya
samādhi-pariṇāmaḥ

7. These three (dhāranā, dhyāna and samādhi) affect
more directly than the five previously described paths;
(yama, niyama, āsana, prānāyāma and pratyāhāra).

Once samyama is established, the state of consciousness
yoga can be experienced, while yama, niyama, āsana,
prānāyāma, and pratyāhāra are different paths that can
lead to yoga.

8. But even these three (dhāranā, dhyāna and samādhi)
are inferior to the highest level of samādhi.

Samādhi can be experienced as inner peace and tranquility, but absent of sensory experiences. The highest
state of samādhi occurs when awareness is completely
absorbed in Consciousness. From this samādhi there is
no return back to the ignorance where the mind rules
and where identification with the mind takes place.

9. Nirodha parināmah is a state where awareness is
present in ongoing sensory experiences and in vanishing
sensory experiences, thus to be established in silence and
stillness without sensory sensations.

Nirodha parināmah is the transition from being bound
by sensory senses to being an observer of what is happening in the present.

*10. Then a flowing, calm and peaceful state of awareness
arises.*

*When sensory experiences cease, there are no conflicts,
no resistance, and no duality. When all resistance is
gone, a flow of peace, well-being and silence is experienced.*

*11. The state of consciousness samādhi parināmah is
characterized by the experience of unity. All disturbances are then gone.*

*Samādhi parināmah means that all division and duality
is gone and has been replaced by wholeness and unity.*

ततः पुनः शान्तोदितौ तुल्यप्रत्ययौ
चित्तस्यैकाग्रतापरिणामः॥१२॥

12. Tataḥ punaḥ śāntoditau tulya-pratyayau cit-
tasyaikāgratā-pariṇāmaḥ

एतेन भूतेन्द्रियेषु धर्मलक्षणावस्थापरिणामा
व्याख्याताः॥१३॥

13. Etena bhūtendriyeṣu dharma-lakṣaṇā-vast-
hā-pariṇāmā vyākhyātāḥ

शान्तोदिताव्यपदेश्यधर्मानुपाती धर्मी॥१४॥

14. Śāntoditāvyapadeśya-dharmānupātī dharmī

क्रमान्यत्वं परिणामान्यत्वे हेतुः॥१५॥

15. Kramānyatvaṁ pariṇāmānyatve hetuḥ

12. *Ekāgratā parināma is a state of awareness which
means that the conscious presence is bound to a
constant flow of sensory sensations both from the past
and from the present.*

*As long as this state of awareness is present, it means a
constant bond to the mind and sensory sensations both
from the past, present and future.*

13. *The state of awareness changes depending on characteristics, character, and the function of the body and the
sense organs.*

*How awareness perceives life in the present depends,
among other things, on the body and the function and
properties of the mind.*

14. *All manifested objects are characterized by the fact
that they change and have a past, a being in the present,
and a future.*

*Objects in space and time are constantly changing and
are bound to the principle of the maintenance and
degradation of creation.*

15. *The cause of the changes are the laws of nature that
govern evolution.*

The relative manifested existence is governed by certain given laws of nature.

In the following sutras, Patanjali gives various suggestions on how it is possible to influence the laws of nature and the manifested relative existence, and how it is possible to obtain so-called, siddhis (occult forces). Some yogis consider it reprehensible to use these siddhis as they draw attention to the mind and ego and away from the divine Consciousness. In sutra 38, Patanjali says that they are obstacles to achieving samādhi.

परिणामत्रयसंयमादतीतानागतज्ञानम्॥१६॥

16. Pariṇāma-traya-saṁyamād atītānāgata-jñānam

शब्दार्थप्रत्ययानामितरेतराध्यासात्सङ्करसत्तत्प्रवि
भागसंयमात्सर्वभूतरुतज्ञानम्॥१७॥

17. Śabdārtha-pratyayānām itaretarādhyāsāt
samkaras tat-pravibhāga-saṁyamāt sarva-bhū-
ta-ruta-jñānam

संस्कारसाक्षात्करणात्पूर्वजातिज्ञानम्॥१८॥

18. Saṁskāra-sākṣātkaraṇāt pūrva-jātijñānam

प्रत्ययस्य परचित्तिज्ञानम्॥१९॥

19. Pratyayasya para-citta-jñānam

न च तत्सालम्बनं तस्यावषियीभूतत्वात्॥२०॥

20. Na ca tat sālambanaṁ tasyāviṣayī-bhū-tatvāt

कायरूपसंयमात्तद्ग्राह्यशक्तिस्तम्भे चक्षुःप्रकाशास
म्प्रयोगेऽन्तर्धानम्॥२१॥

21. Kāya-rūpa-saṁyamāt tad-grāhya-śakti-stam-
bhe cakṣuḥ-prakāśāsamprayoge ’ntardhānam

एतेन शदाद्यतधार्नमुक्तमः ॥ २२॥

22. Etena śabdādy antardhānam uktamḥ

16. *By practicing the samyama on the three changing states (nirodha, samādhi and ekāgrata), knowledge of the past and of the future can be obtained.*

17. *A sound, its meaning, and idea are mixed. By making samyama on each part separately, this results in that, the sounds of all living beings can be understood.*

18. *By performing samyama on past experiences, knowledge of past lives can be obtained.*

19. *Doing samyama on mental images that arise consciously can provide knowledge about the minds of others.*

20. *The purpose of practicing samyama on the minds of others is not the content but the quality and feeling experienced.*

21. *By making samyama on the shape of a body, the contact between an observer's eye and the light of the body can be broken and it can then become invisible.*

22. *The result is also that sounds etc., cease to be heard.*

सोपक्रमं निरुपक्रमं च कर्म
तत्संयमादपरान्तज्ञानमरिष्टेभ्यो वा॥२२॥
23. Sopakramaṁ nirupakramaṁ ca karma
tat-saṁyamād aparānta-jñānam ariṣṭebhyo vā

मैत्र्यादिषु बलानि॥२३॥
24. Maitryādiṣu balāni

बलेषु हस्तिबलादीनि॥२४॥
25. Baleṣu hasti-balādīni

प्रवृत्त्यालोकन्यासात्सूक्ष्मव्यवहतिविप्रकृष्टज्ञानम्॥२५॥
26. Pravṛtty-āloka-nyāsāt sūkṣma-vyavahita-vi-
prakṛṣṭa-jñānam

भुवनज्ञानं सूर्ये संयमात्॥२६॥
27. Bhuvana-jñānaṁ sūrye saṁyamāt

चन्द्रे तारायूहज्ञानम्॥२७॥
28. Candre tārā-vyūha-jñānam

23. By performing samyama on two kinds of karma; the active and the dormant, the time of the moment of death can be experienced.

24. Practicing samyama in kindness, compassion, and happiness can mean that these qualities are obtained.

25. By practicing the samyama on the strength of an elephant, such strength can be obtained.

26. To practice samyama on the inner light, knowledge of the subtle, the hidden, and the distant object can be obtained.

27. By doing samyama on the sun, knowledge of the solar system can be obtained.

28. Practicing samyama on the moon, can provide knowledge of star systems.

ध्रुवे तद्गतिज्ञानम्॥२८॥

29. Dhruve tad-gati-jñānam

नाभिचक्रे कायव्यूहज्ञानम्॥२९॥

30. Nābhi-cakre kāya-vyūhajñānam

कण्ठकूपे क्षुत्पिपासानिवृत्तिः॥३०॥

31. Kaṇṭha-kūpe kṣut-pipāsā-nivṛttiḥ

कूर्मनाड्यां स्थैर्यम्॥३१॥

32. Kūrma-nāḍyāṁ sthairyam

मूर्धज्योतिषि सिद्धदर्शनम्॥३२॥

33. Mūrdha-jyotiṣi siddha-darśanam

प्रातिभाद्वा सर्वम्॥३३॥

34. Prātibhād vā sarvam

हृदये चित्तसंवित्॥३४॥

35. Hṛdaye citta-saṁvit

29. By practicing the samyama on the pole star, this gives knowledge of the movements of the stars.

30. To make samyama on the navel, knowledge of the structure of the body can be obtained.

31. Through samyama on the trachea, hunger and thirst can be quenched.

32. Practicing samyama on the bronchial tubes (kūr-ma-nādi) provides silence.

33. By practicing samyama on the light in the head enlightened persons (siddhas) may be experienced.

34. Practicing samyama on intuition (prātibhā), means that everything can be understood.

35. By practicing samyama on the heart, knowledge of the mind can be obtained.

सत्त्वपुरुषयोरत्यन्तासङ्कीर्णयोः प्रत्ययाविशेषो
भोगः परार्थत्वात्स्वार्थसंयमात्पुरुषज्ञानम्॥३५॥
36. Sattva-puruṣayor atyantāsaṅkīrṇayoḥ praty-
ayāviśeṣo bhogaḥ parārthat svārtha saṁyamāt
puruṣa-jñānam

ततः प्रातिभश्रावणवेदनादर्शास्वादवार्ता
जायन्ते॥३६॥
37. Tataḥ prātibha-śrāvaṇa-vedanādarśāsvā-
da-vārtā jāyante

ते समाधावुपसर्गा व्युत्थाने सिद्धयः॥३७॥
38. Te samādhāv upasargā vyutthāne siddhayaḥ

बन्धकारणशैथिल्यात्प्रचारसंवेदनाच्च चित्तस्य
परशरीरावेशः॥३८॥
39. Bandha-kāraṇa-śaithilyāt pracāra-saṁvedanāc
ca cittasya para-śarīrāveśaḥ

उदानजयाज्जलपङ्ककण्टकादिष्विवसङ्ग
उत्क्रान्तिश्च॥३९॥
40. Udāna-jayāj jala-paṅka-kaṇṭakādiṣv asaṅga
utkrāntiś ca

36. Being consciously present in the intellectual mind and being consciously present in consciousness are two completely different states of consciousness. By exercising the samyama on the distinction between the intellect and Consciousness (purusa), Consciousness can be experienced.

37. This conscious presence in the consciousness gives the finest hearing, finest feeling, finest sight, finest taste and finest smell.

38. These forces (siddhis) are obstacles to achieving samādi as they draw attention to the mind.

39. When consciousness is unbound and has knowledge of the flow of energy in the body, it is possible to enter someone else's body.

40. By controlling the life energy (udāna) one can walk on water, over swamps or thorns, and at will one can leave the body.

समानजयाज्ज्वलनम्॥४०॥

41. Samāna-jayāj jvalanam

श्रोत्राकाशयोः सम्बन्धसंयमाद्दविृयं श्रोत्रम्॥४१॥

42. Śrotrākāśayoḥ sambandha-saṁyamād divyaṁ
śrotram

कायाकाशयोः सम्बन्धसंयमाल्लघुतूलसमापत्तेश्चाका
शगमनम्॥४२॥

43. Kāyākāśayoḥ sambandha-saṁyamāt lag-
hutūlasamāpatteścākāśagamanam

वहिरिकल्पिता वृत्तिर्मिहावदिेहा ततः
प्रकाशावरणक्षयः॥४३॥

44. Bahir akalpitā vṛttir mahā-videhā tataḥ
prakāśāvaraṇa kṣayaḥ

स्थूलसवरूपसूक्ष्मान्वयार्थवत्त्वसंयमादभूतजयः॥४४॥

45. Sthūla-svarūpa-sūkṣmānvayārthavattva-saṁy-
amād bhūta-jayaḥ

41. *By controlling the energy samāna (located in the solar plexus), the body can radiate light.*

42. *By exercising the samyama on the connection between hearing and ākāśa (ether or space), divine hearing can be obtained.*

43. *Practicing samyama on the connection between the body and ākāśa results in ease as in cotton fiber, and then the body can fly through the air.*

44. *To consciously free oneself from the limitations of the mind is called mahāvidehā, whereby the veil which hinders the light of distinction can be destroyed.*

45. *By samyama on the qualities of the five elements (bhūtas) as the coarse forms, the subtle constituents and their purpose, the elements can be mastered.*

ततोऽणिमादिप्रादुर्भावः
कायसम्पत्तद्धर्मानभिघातश्च ॥४५॥

46. Tato 'ṇimādi-prādurbhāvaḥ kāya-sampat tad
dharmā anabhighātaś ca

रूपलावण्यबलवज्रसंहननत्वानि कायसम्पत् ॥४६॥

47. Rūpa-lāvaṇya-bala-vajra-saṁhananatvāni
kāya-sampat

ग्रहणस्वरूपास्मितान्वयार्थवत्त्वसंयमादिन्द्रियजयः ॥४७॥

48. Grahaṇa-sva-rūpa-āsmitā-anvayārthavatt-
va-saṁyamād indriya-jayaḥ

ततो मनोजवित्वं विकरणभावः प्रधानजयश्च ॥४८॥

49. Tato manojavitvaṁ vikaraṇa-bhāvaḥ pradhā-
na-jayaś ca

सत्त्वपुरुषान्यताख्यातिमात्रस्य सर्वभावाधिष्ठातृत्वं
सर्वज्ञातृत्वं च ॥४९॥

50. Sattva-puruṣānyatā-khyāti-mātrasya sar-
va-bhāvādhiṣṭhātṛtvaṁ sarvajñātṛtvaṁ ca

46. This gives the ability to change the proportions of the body (animā), such as size. This can lead to the perfection of body and mind.

47. Perfection of the body means beauty, charisma, strength and a firmness like a diamond.

48. Through samyama of the sense organs, their character, quality and purpose as well as the ego (asmitā), a conscious presence arises in the mind and thereby control is gained over it.

49. Through control of the mind, awareness is obtained that is not dependent on body and mind, awareness of the ultimate cause in nature (pradhāna) is established.

50. By performing samyama on the distinction between intellect and consciousness (purusa) omnipotence and omniscience are obtained.

तद्वैराग्यादपि दोषबीजक्षये कैवल्यम्॥५०॥

51. Tad-vairāgyād api doṣa-bīja-kṣaye kaivalyam

स्थान्युपनिमन्त्रणे सङ्गस्मयाकरणं
पुनरनिष्टप्रसङ्गात्॥५१॥

52. Sthāny-upanimantraṇe saṅga smayā-karaṇaṁ
punar aniṣṭa-prasaṅgāt

क्षणतत्क्रमयोः संयमाद्वविकजं ज्ञानम्॥५२॥

53. Kṣaṇa-tat-kramayoḥ saṁyamād vivekajaṁ
jñānam

जातलिक्षणदेशैरन्यतानवच्छेदात्तुल्यययोस्ततः
परतपित्ततिः॥५३॥

54. Jāti-lakṣaṇa-deśair anyatānavacchedāt tulyay-
os tataḥ pratipattiḥ

तारकं सर्ववषियं सर्वथावषियमक्रमं चेति वविकजं
ज्ञानम्॥५४॥

55. Tārakaṁ sarva viṣayaṁ sarvathā viṣayam
akramaṁ ceti vivekajaṁ jñānam

सत्त्वपुरुषयोः शुद्धसिाम्ये कैवल्यमति॥५५॥

56. Sattva-puruṣayoḥ śuddhi sāmye kaivalyam

51. *To renounce these forces means that awareness leaves the seed to the bonds of karma to be liberated and enlightened (kaivalya).*

52. *When heavenly beings are tempting, temptation can lead to false pride and flattery, leading to a fall and to unconsciousness.*

53. *By performing samyamā on the present, knowledge can be obtained through distinction.*

To be consciously present in the now means to be in the now and in eternity at the same time. Being rooted in this level of consciousness means being able to distinguish reality from the illusion, as reality only exists in the present.

54. *By applying this knowledge, two similar objects can be distinguished from each other.*

55. *The highest knowledge arises when there is presence in Consciousness. This knowledge includes everything that can be experienced from the past, in the present, and in the future, and is unbound to time and space.*

56. *Enlightenment (kaivalyam) arises through purification (śuddhi), so that awareness can be present in Consciousness (purusa).*

*When mental and physical barriers do not receive atten-
tion, awareness can become present in Consciousness.*

Chapter 4

KAIVALYA PADA

Enlightenment

जन्मौषधमिन्त्ररतपःसमाधजिाः सदि्धयः॥१॥

1. Janmauṣadhi-mantra-tapaḥ-samādhi-jāḥ siddhayaḥ

जात्यन्तरपरणिामः प्रकृत्यापूरात्॥२॥

2. Jāty-antara-pariṇāmaḥ prakṛty-āpūrāt

नमित्तिमप्रयोजकं प्रकृतीनां वरणभेदस्तु ततः
क्षेत्ररकिवत्॥३॥

3. Nimittam aprayojakaṁ prakṛtīnāṁ varaṇa-bhe-
das tu tataḥ kṣetrikavat

नरि्माणचति्तान्यस्मतिामात्रात्॥४॥

4. Nirmāṇa-cittāny asmitā-mātrāt

प्रवृत्तभिदे प्रयोजकं चति्तमेकमनेकेषाम्॥५॥

5. Pravṛtti-bhede prayojakaṁ cittam ekam ane-
keṣām

तत्र ध्यानजमनाशयम्॥६॥

6. Tatra dhyānajam anāśayam

1. The supernatural abilities (siddhis) can be innate or they can arise through drugs (ausadhi), by clean life and abstinence (tapas), by using mantras or being in samādhi.

In Chapter 3, Patanjali describes how siddhis can arise by practicing samyama. They can also occur spontaneously for any of the reasons stated in this sutra.

2. The transition from one level of consciousness to another takes place quite naturally and spontaneously when a level of consciousness has fulfilled its function. In the same way that H2O can change and be liquid water, solid ice or volatile steam, consciousness can change over a period of life.

3. Actions that lead to change are not the cause of the change, they only remove the obstacles to the changes of nature (praktī), such as a farmer who changes the natural flow of water by removing obstacles to the water. At a relative level, there is a constant, ever ongoing change. It is praktī (the relative nature) that is the cause of this constant change. To be only consciously present in this change means to be constantly anchored in the relative. By shifting the focus of attention to the absolute Consciousness, a change can take place. Changing the focus of attention then means a shift from one level of consciousness to another. Actions that remove obstacles can be the practice of pranayama, yoga asanas or meditation which can remove mental imbalance or bodily tensions, which means that the natural flow of life becomes reality in the present.

4. All sensory sensations arise through presence and identification with the ego.

5. All relative mental sensory sensations originate in the nature of the mind (pravritti).

6. Only those mental sensations that arise spontaneously during meditation are free from desire.

कर्माशुक्लाकृष्णं योगनिस्त्रिविधमितरेषाम् ॥७॥

7. Karmāśuklākṛṣṇaṁ yoginas tri-vidham itareṣām

ततस्तद्विपाकानुगुणानामेवाभिव्यक्तिर्वासनानाम् ॥८॥

8. Tatas tad-vipākānuguṇānām evābhivyaktir
vāsanānām

जातिदेशकालव्यवहितानामप्यानन्तर्यं
स्मृतिसंस्कारयोरेकरूपत्वात् ॥९॥

9. Jāti-deśa-kāla-vyavahitānām apy ānantar-yaṁ
smṛti-saṁskārayor ekarūpatvāt

तासामनादित्वं चाशिषो नित्यत्वात् ॥१०॥

10. Tāsām anāditvaṁ cāśiṣo nityatvāt

हेतुफलाश्रयालम्बनैः सङ्गृहीतत्वादेषामभावे
तदभावः ॥११॥

11. Hetu-phalāśrayālambanaiḥ saṅgṛhītatvād eṣām
abhāve tad-abhāvaḥ

अतीतानागतं स्वरूपतोऽस्त्यध्वभेदाद्धर्माणाम् ॥१२॥

12. Atītānāgataṁ svarūpato 'sty adhva-bhedād
dharmāṇām

*7. A yogi's karma is neither dark (unclean) nor light
(pure), like the karma of others which is threefold, dark,
light or mixed.*

*Karma nurtures and teaches through sowing and
reaping in the path of life. A yogi who is established and
rooted in Consciousness does not need this teaching of
life and is therefore independent of karma.*

*8. When the circumstances are suitable for threefold
karma, karma is manifested, which then bears fruit.*

*9. Through memories and experiences, the cause and
effect of karma remain regardless of life situation, time
and space.*

*10. The desire to live has always existed and therefore
life is eternal.*

*It is not always possible to refer to the fact that you have
always been alive, this is often because the memory
cannot provide information about this. But just because
you can not remember and be aware of your first year
of life, you do not have to deny that you have been alive
this year.*

*11. As long as the mind is bound to the cause and effect
of karma, awareness is bound to the mind.*

*12. The past and the future exist only as mental sensa-
tions which are distinguished by different characteristics
and qualities.*

ते व्यक्तसूक्ष्मा गुणात्मानः ॥१३॥

13. Te vyakta-sūkṣmā guṇātmānaḥ

परिणामैकत्वाद्वस्तुतत्त्वम् ॥१४॥

14. Pariṇāmaikatvād vastu-tattvam

वस्तुसाम्ये चित्तभेदात्तयोर्विभिक्तः पन्थाः ॥१५॥

15. Vastu-sāmye citta-bhedāt tayor vibhaktaḥ
    panthāḥ

न चैकचित्ततन्त्रं वस्तु तदप्रमाणकं तदा किं
स्यात् ॥१६॥

16. Na caika-citta-tantraṁ vastu tad-apramā-ṇa-
    kaṁ tadā kiṁ syāt

तदुपरागापेक्षित्वाच्चित्तस्य वस्तु
ज्ञाताज्ञातम् ॥१७॥

17. Tad-uparāgāpekṣitvāc cittasya vastu
    jñātājñātam

सदा ज्ञाताश्चित्तवृत्तयस्तत्प्रभोः
पुरुषस्यापरिणामित्वात् ॥१८॥

18. Sadā jñātāś citta-vṛttayas tat-prabhoḥ
    puruṣasyāpariṇāmitvāt

13. They can be manifest or unmanifest and have different characteristics and qualities (gunās).

14. The unique state of an object in the present depends on the influence of the three gunās and this applies to all relative existence.

15. Sensory perceptions are experienced differently depending on the level of consciousness that prevails.

16. An object is not dependent on a single mind, if so, what would happen if an object is not experienced by this mind?

Although the sensory perceptions of an object are mental experiences, an object has its own existence whether it is experienced or not.

17. An object can only be experienced if the sense perception is present for consciousness.

If consciousness is rooted in thoughts other than what is happening in the present, the experience of an object can be lost.

18. All changes in the mind are witnessed by Consciousness which is constantly the unchanging observer.

The changing relative existence can only be witnessed by the unchanging eternal Consciousness.

न तत्स्वाभासं दृश्यत्वात्॥१९॥

19. Na tat svābhāsaṁ dṛśyatvāt

एकसमये चोभयानवधारणम्॥२०॥

20. Eka-samaye cobhayānavadhāraṇam

चित्तान्तरदृश्ये बुद्धिबुद्धेरतिप्रसङ्गः
स्मृतिसङ्करश्च॥२१॥

21. Cittāntara-dṛśye buddhi-buddher ati-pra-
saṅgaḥ smṛti-saṅkaraś ca

चितेरप्रतिसङ्क्रमायास्तदाकारापत्तौ
स्वबुद्धिसंवेदनम्॥२२॥

22. Citerapratisaṅkramāyāstadākārāpattau sva-
buddhisaṁvedanam

द्रष्टृदृश्योपरक्तं चित्तं सर्वार्थम्॥२३॥

23. Draṣṭṛdṛśyoparaktaṁ cittaṁ sarvārtham

*19. The mind is not self-enlightened, although it is
perceptible.*

*Like the moon which does not shine by itself but by the
rays of the sun, the mind is illuminated only by Consciousness. The mind is a tool for sensory sensations to
become aware.*

*20. Since the mind is not self-enlightened, it cannot be
consciously present in both the senses and in Consciousness at the same time.*

*Being anchored in the mind and consciously present
in the sensory sensations does not mean simultaneous
presence in Consciousness. Only by being consciously
anchored in the Consciousness can conscious presence
arise in both the mind and Consciousness at the same
time.*

*21. If the mind could be experienced by another mind,
confusion would arise as to which mind belongs to
memories and sensory perceptions.*

*At the level of relative existence, it is necessary that each
mind is delimited and limited to an individual consciousness, so that the life situation does not become chaotic
and incomprehensible.*

22. Consciousness is immutable, but when awareness identifies with the changing intellect (buddhi) and the senses of the mind it loses contact with Consciousness.

23. Awareness is colored by both the observing absolute Consciousness and the observed relative objects.

तदसङ्ख्येयवासनाभिश्चित्रमपि परार्थं
संहत्यकारित्वात् ॥२४॥

24. Tadasaṅkhyeyavāsanābhiścitramapi parārtham
saṁhatyakāritvāt

विशेषदर्शिनि आत्मभावभावनाविनिवृत्तिः ॥२५॥

25. Viśeṣa-darśina ātma-bhāva-bhāvanā-vinivṛttiḥ

तदा विविकनिम्निङ्कैवल्यप्राग्भारञ्चित्तम् ॥२६॥

26. Tadā viveka-nimnaṁ kaivalya-prāg-bhāraṁ
cittam

तच्छिद्रेषु प्रत्ययान्तराणि संस्कारेभ्यः ॥२७॥

27. Tac chidreṣu pratyayāntarāṇi saṁskārebhyaḥ

हानमेषां क्लेशवदुक्तम् ॥२८॥

28. Hānameṣāṁ kleśavad uktam

प्रसङ्ख्यानेऽप्यकुसीदस्य सर्वथा
विविकख्यातेर्धर्ममेघः समाधिः ॥२९॥

29. Prasaṅkhyāne 'py akusīdasya sarvathā vive-
ka-khyāter dharma-meghaḥ samādhiḥ

24. Awareness affected by various senses and desires (vāsanās) is dependent on Consciousness and its higher purpose.

25. He who is consciously present in Consciousness ceases to seek his identity in sensory perceptions in the mind and ego.

26. Then, when awareness has the ability to distinguish and observe (viveka) the sensory sensations (cittam), absolute freedom (kaivalya) can arise.

27. When awareness does not have the ability to distinguish and observe thoughts and feelings from past, experiences will affect awareness.

There is an individual bank of experiences that lies latent and is activated by memory and becomes conscious with the help of thoughts and feelings. If awareness is not consciously present and can observe and distinguish in the present, the past experiences will automatically be activated to help with appropriate information from the past.

28. These can be removed in the same way as other disorders that lead to suffering (kleśas).

Some thoughts and feelings from past experiences can be an obstacle to presence in Consciousness and the state of yoga. Therefore, their influence over awareness must be overcome and removed.

29. Then this constant, selfless, distinctive, state of consciousness has resulted in the ultimate supreme state where awareness "from a cloud giving rain in the form of heavenly virtue and grace "dharma meghah samādhih".

When awareness is present in consciousness, this state gives total satisfaction and then there is no need to seek more satisfaction. That the mind should try to intellectually suffocate obstacles that arise in the form of thoughts and feelings is ineffective when they are back sooner or later. That is, awareness as through "a rain in the form of heavenly virtue and grace" (dharma meghah samādhih) that can do this and bring awareness in Consciousness. The mind can be helpful to the awareness by being cooperative and e.g. apply one or more of the eightfold paths; yama, niyama, asanas, pranayama, pratyahara, dharana, dhyana and samadhi, but it is the grace of God that ultimately establishes the consciousness of Samadhi.

ततः क्लेशकर्मनिवृत्तिः॥३०॥

30. Tataḥ kleśa-karma-nivṛttiḥ

तदा सर्वावरणमलापेतस्य ज्ञानस्यानन्त्याज्ज्ञेयम
ल्पम्॥३१॥

31. Tadā sarvāvaraṇa-malāpetasya jñānasyā-nan-
tyāj jñeyam alpam

ततः कृतार्थानां परिणामक्रमसमाप्तिर्गुणानाम्॥३२॥

32. Tataḥ kṛtārthānāṁ pariṇāma-krama-samāptir
guṇānām

क्षणप्रतियोगी परिणामापरान्तनिर्ग्राह्यः
क्रमः॥३३॥

33. Kṣaṇa-pratiyogī pariṇāmāparānta-nirgrāhyaḥ
kramaḥ

पुरुषार्थशून्यानां गुणानां प्रतिप्रसवः कैवल्यं
स्वरूपप्रतिष्ठा वा चितिशक्तिरिति॥३४॥

34. Puruṣārtha-śūnyānāṁ guṇānāṁ pratiprasavaḥ
kaivalyaṁ svarūpa-pratiṣṭhā vā citi-śakter iti

30. Then all disturbances and obstacles cease, as well as the effects of karma that cause suffering.

31. When distractions and obstacles have been removed, knowledge emerges that cannot be compared with the limited intellectual knowledge of the mind.

Different types of disturbances and obstacles from the experience bank then no longer fill any function. Of course, useful experiences from the past can be used in the present.

32. Once the state of dharma meghah samādhi is established, the three gunas (tamas, rajas and sattva) have fulfilled their duties.

The three gunas have tasks to perform and when that is done, they have finished playing their roles in the arena of the mind.

33. Kramah is an element of the constant change that takes place in the eternal present and can be experienced when the three gunas are transformed.

In parallel with the constant change in the relative existence, there is the absolute eternal immutable being. The changing existence can only be experienced by its opposite, the unchanging being.

34. Kaivalya is the state of consciousness that arises when the three gunas no longer affect, as they no longer have any purpose to fill. Then awareness is present in the real state of consciousness which is pure Consciousness.

Postscript

Patanjalis Yoga Sutras can be seen as a handbook in describing the real and the illusory existence. Ie., to be present in the eternal absolute pure Consciousness and to be bound by the perishable relative existence. Patanjali's sutras are characterized by nondualism, ie., that there is no contradiction between the absolute Consciousness and the relative mind and ego. There is only one Consciousness at the absolute level, only the degree of awareness is different at the relative level.

The basic purpose is not to create a belief system with intellectual interpretations but to provide an accurate description of the yogic process that can be verified through one's own experiences of Yoga and the state of consciousness Samadhi. It is possible to look at the sutras from a scientific philosophical perspective. It then becomes a dualistic view whose purpose is to do scientific research, investigate and compare the sutras, not to transcend the mind to be present in Yoga, Samadhi.

Ultimately, it is the Yoga and state of consciousness, Samadhi that provides confirmation and contributes to an identity shift from bondage in mind to presence in Consciousness . The change of identity takes place when there is sufficient maturity for it. This does not mean that the intellect and senses disappear but that they are refined.

With Ashtanga Yoga, Patanjali describes eight different tools to help establish awareness in Consciousness that is constantly present and eternal. The purpose of the sutras and the aids he proposes is that constant presence in Consciousness, in Yoga, shall be established.

By applying samyama to Patanjali's sutras, qualities such as kindness, compassion, humility, and selflessness can be established and inner peace, happiness, and harmony can arise in life.

Tat Tvam Asi - Thou art That.

Om shanti shanti shanti!

HATHA YOGA
Pradipika

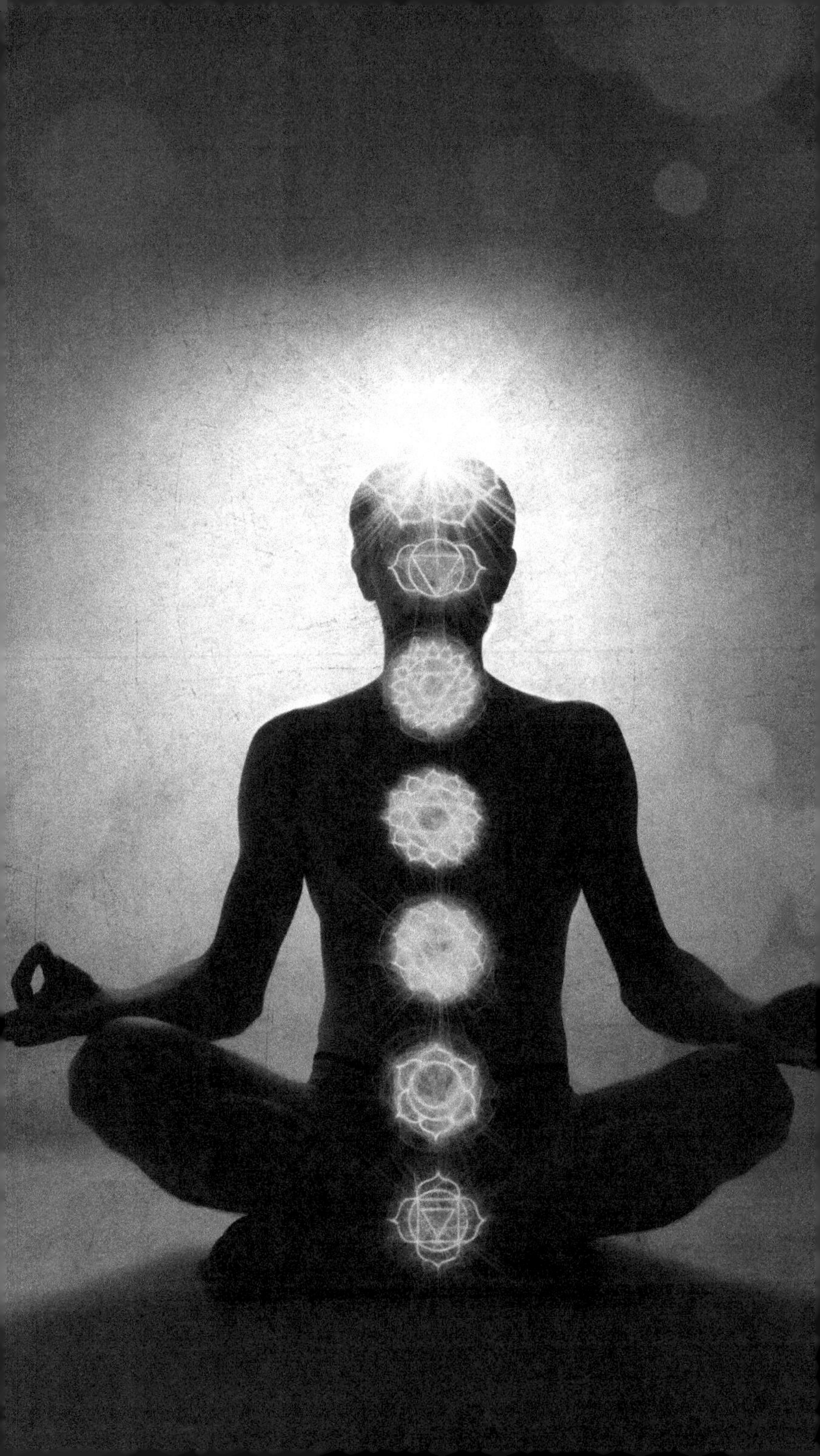

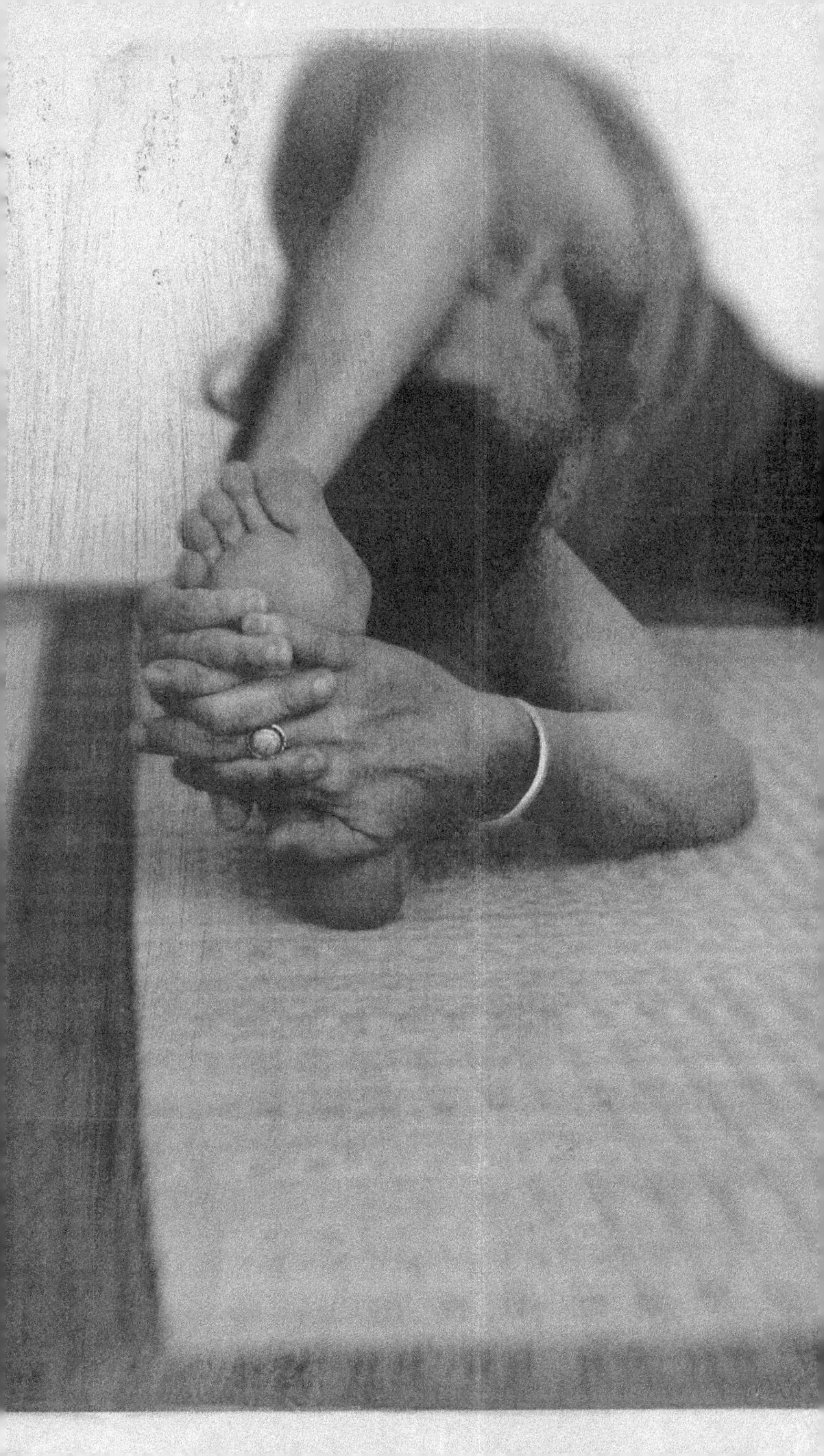

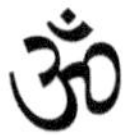

"As one opens the door with a key, so the yogi should
open the gate to liberation with the kundalini.

The great goddess sleeps, closing with her mouth,
the opening through which one can ascend to the
Brahmarandhra...
to that place where there is neither pain nor suffering.

The kundalini sleeps above the kanda...
she gives liberation to the yogi and bondage to the fool.

He who knows kundalini, knows yoga.

The kundalini, it is said, is coiled like a serpent.
He who can induce her to move is liberated."

Hatha Yoga Pradipika v. 105-111.

Introduction

Hatha Yoga Pradipika.

Is the No.1 most read book about yoga besides Patanjalis Yogasutras. The Hatha Yoga Pradipika, along with the Gheranda-Samhita (1650), is one of the most detailed manuals describing the techniques of Hatha Yoga. The book is the hatha yoga text that has historically been studied within yoga teacher training programmes, alongside texts on classical yoga such as Patanjali's Yoga Sutras.

The HYP is a medieval yoga text, dating from about the 15th or 16th century, and is as much about Tantra as about Yoga. It was compiled by Swātmārama. It´s name means "special (pra) light (dipika) on forceful (hatha) yoga". It is much later in date than the Yoga Sutras, and provides details of Hatha Yoga techniques which the Yoga Sutras don't touch on. But there are also occasional sutras which touch on familiar concerns (for example, compare HYP 4.23 with YS 1.2). It is just about yoga practice, as contrasted with the Bhagavad Gītā, which is about how to live in the everyday world.

The word "hatha" requires a little comment. The concept is that we live in an energy field; energy is behind all action. The energy field that we live in normally extends 4 fingers-breadth beyond the body, and it is possible also in a healthy person to achieve a situation in which the energy is concentrated inside the body. In an unhealthy person the energy dissipates further. There are blockages in an unhealthy person that makes it impossible to concentrate one's energy properly, and techniques such as nadi śodhana are used to open the channels and improve the flow of energy.

There is in fact a whole complex of energy channels or nādī within the body, of which there are 11 primary nadi, coming from a central hub (kanda) located in the lower abdomen, and branching out into many others (traditionally, 72,000).

There are 10 nadi associated with perception and action:

eyes (sight)

tongue (speech)

ears (hearing)

fingers & thumbs (grasping)

tongue (taste)

big toes (locomotion)

skin (feeling)

bladder & anus (excretion)

nostrils (smell)

sex organs (generation)

If the quality of the nadi is poor, the quality of perception and action is also poor.

There is one more nadi, the susumna, which instead of flowing out, flows in, linking us to the inner world. It runs from the kanda to the base of the spine then to the top of the head. There are two processes in energy, ha and tha, which flow through the pingala and ida channels (or nādī) respectively, and then unite to flow into susumna. Usually it is not possible for energy to flow into susumna because of a blockage at the base of the spine. The practice of Hatha Yoga tries to create a state of breakthrough allowing energy to flow into susumna, bringing with it a stable state of mind. The Hatha Yoga Pradipika teaches techniques that allow this state to be achieved.

The difference between the Hatha Yoga of the Hatha Yoga Pradipika and the Raja Yoga of the Yoga Sutras is that Hatha Yoga uses prana as a primary working tool, whereas Raja Yoga uses the mind as its primary working tool. These days very few people are able to practice Hatha Yoga sufficiently strongly for it to work properly.

The key ideas in the text are:

Chapter 1 – āsana: used to stimulate energy (prana);
Chapter 2 – prānāyāma: used to contain/condense energy;
Chapter 3 – mudrā: used to direct energy;
Chapter 4 – dhyāna: used to integrate and merge energy.

Chapter Summaries:

CHAPTER 1: Asanas.
1-11 Introduction.
Hatha yoga "shines forth as a stairway to raja yoga" (1); is "the greatest secret of the yogis who wish to attain perfection".
12-16 Conditions for practice.
The "hermitage" described (12-14); obstacles and supports (15-16). The ten yama and ten niyama in sutras 16ii and 16iii are apparently later additions to the text; hatha yoga does not in fact place much emphasis on them.

17-56 Āsana.

The role of āsana is to develop steadiness of body and mind, flexibility of the limbs; sequence for practice is āsana → prāṇāyāma → mudrā → meditation (56).

57-63 Diet and Restrictions.

Mitāhāra – appropriate food (57, 62-63); food to avoid (58-59); other things to avoid (60-61).

64-67 Conclusion.

Importance of practical application emphasised (64-66); hatha yoga leads to Raja Yoga (67).

CHAPTER 2: Prāṇāyāmas.

1-3 Breath and mind.

First make the body steady, then bring steadiness to prāṇa (1); when prāṇa moves, citta moves (2).

4-5 Nāḍī and malā.

Nadīs must be purified so that prāṇa can flow.

6-20 Practice guidelines.

Practice daily (6); nadi śodhana (7-12); milk and ghee important foods (14); negative effects of inappropriate practice (15-17); indications of purification (18-20).

21-36 The Śat Karma (cleansing techniques).

These should be practised only by persons with kapha imbalance (21).

37-74 Prāṇāyāma.

Some teachers say prāṇāyāma alone is enough to cleanse the system (37); prāṇāyāma purifies the nāḍīs and chakras, and opens the door to suśumna (41); manon-

mani – mind devoid of thought (42); eight types of kumbhaka (43-70); three processes of prānāyāma (71-74); two processes of kumbhaka (72-74).

75-77 Kundalini and Raja Yoga.

By practising kumbhaka, kundalini is aroused and suśumna is freed of obstacles (75); both hatha and raja yoga are essential for perfection (samādhi) (76).

78 Eight signs of perfection.

lean body, bright face, strong voice, clear eyes, no disease, control of semen, active digestive fire, purification of nādis.

CHAPTER 3: Mudrās.

1-2 Kundalini.

Kundalini the support of all yoga practices.

3-5 Susumnā.

When kundalini awakens, susumnā becomes pathway of prāna (3); the "goddess sleeping at Brahma's door" can be aroused by performing mudrā.

6-103 Ten mudrās described.

10-18 maha mudra.

19-25 maha bandha.

26-29 maha vedha.

30-31 when to perform these three.

32-54 khechari mudra.

55-60 uddiyana bandha.

61-69 mula bandha.

70-73 jalandhara bandha.

74-77 comments on the three bandhas.

78-82 viparita karani.

83-91 vajroli mudra.

92-95 sahajoli mudra.

96-103 maroli mudra.

104-124 Kundalini.

Kundalini is coiled like a snake(108), 3½ times, at base of susumnā; you have to awaken the snake (111) [like getting rid of a snake in a tree by either hitting the tree with a stick or lighting a fire under it]; this moves kundalini so that it is drawn up into susumnā a little way (117), thus allowing prāna to enter susumnā (118). Best way to do this is to practise bhastrika with kumbhaka (122); other than arousing kundalini, the other way to purify the nadis including susumnā is regular practice of āsana, prānāyāma, mudrā and concentration (124).

125-127 Importance of mental attitude.

Prānāyāma should be practised with a focused mind.

128-130 Conclusion.

CHAPTER 4: Samādhi.

1-9 Samādhi.

Mind and ātman come together in samādhi.

10-29 Prāna.

When prāna flows in susumnā, the mind is blank (12); as well as prāna, air and fire enter suśumnā (19); when mind is still, prāna is suspended, when prāna is suspen-

ded, mind is still (23); if they are controlled, moksa (liberation) is attained (25); this brings steadiness to the body (28).

30-34 Laya (dissolution)

Definition of laya (31).

35-37 Śambhavi mudra (eyebrow centre gazing).

38-47 Khecari.

48 Tūrya.

This "fourth state" is one in which the mind is quiescent.

49-53 Yoga Nidrā.

This is the state in which the conscious mind subsides but awareness remains. It's like a pot filled with space (50).

54-63 Samādhi.

64-102 Nāda.

The sound created by the union of Śiva and Śakti.

Four stages of yoga practice (69-77).

Raja yoga (78-79).

Modern research.

The Hatha Yoga Pradipika is the hatha yoga text that has historically been studied within yoga teacher training programmes, alongside texts on classical yoga such as Patanjali's Yoga Sutras. In the twenty-first century, research on the history of yoga has led to a more developed understanding of hatha yoga's origins.

James Mallinson has studied the origins of hatha yoga in classic yoga texts such as the Khecarīvidyā. He has identified eight works of early hatha yoga that may have contributed to its official formation in the Hatha Yoga Pradipika. This has stimulated further research into understanding the formation of hatha yoga.

Jason Birch has investigated the role of the Hatha Yoga Pradīpikā in popularizing an interpretation of the Sanskrit word hatha. The text drew from classic texts on different systems of yoga, and Svātmārāma grouped what he had found under the generic term "hatha yoga". Examining Buddhist tantric commentaries and earlier medieval yoga texts, Birch found that the adverbial uses of the word suggested that it meant "force", rather than "the metaphysical explanation proposed in the 14th century Yogabīja of uniting the sun (ha) and moon (tha.

The Hatha Yoga Pradipika is also an ocean of secret/hidden knowledge.

Seeker. Listen to this vers:

*"As one opens the door with a key, so the yogi should
open the gate to liberation with the kundalini.*

*The great goddess sleeps, closing with her mouth,
the opening through which one can ascend to the Brahmarandhra…
to that place where there is neither pain nor suffering.*

*The kundalini sleeps above the kanda…
she gives liberation to the yogi and bondage to the fool.*

He who knows kundalini, knows yoga.

*The kundalini, it is said, is coiled like a serpent.
He who can induce her to move is liberated."*

Hatha Yoga Pradipika v. 105-111.

Om Sri Durgayai Namah

*Remebering we are one. Be always united with the force
of the universe. She will take care about you but not for
free. Remember this.*

Yogi Shreyananda Natha

Chapter 1

ASANAS

Prathamopadeśah

1.) śrī-ādi-nāthāya namo|astu tasmai yeno-padiṣhṭā haṭha-yogha-vidyā | vibhrājate pronnata-rāja-yogham āroḍhumichchorad-hirohiṇīva

Salutations to Shiva, who taught the science of Hatha Yoga. It is the aspirant's stairway to the heights of Raja Yoga.

2.) praṇamya śrī-ghuruṃ nāthaṃ svātmārā-meṇa yoghinā | kevalaṃ rāja-yoghāya haṭha-vidyopadiśyate

Yogi Svatmarama, after saluting the Lord and guru, explains the science of Hatha for one reason – Raja Yoga.

3.) bhrāntyā bahumata-dhvānte rāja-yogha-majānatām | haṭha-pradīpikāṃ dhatte svāt-mārāmaḥ kṛpākaraḥ

For those ignorant of Raja Yoga, wandering in the dark-ness of too many opinions, compassionate Svatmarama gives the light of Hatha.

**4.) haṭha-vidyāṃ hi matsyendra-ghorakṣhā-
dyā vijānate | svātmārāmo|athavā yoghī
jānīte tat-prasādataḥ**

*Matsyendra, Goraksha, and others know well the science
of Hatha. By their grace, Yogi Svatmarama also knows
it.*

*The following Siddhas (masters) are said to have existed
in former times. Guru–shishya means "succession from
Guru to disciple". Paramparā literally means an unin-
terrupted row or series, order, succession, continuation,
mediation, tradition.*

**5.) śrī-ādinātha-matsyendra-śāvarānan-
da-bhairavāḥ | chaurangghī-mīna-gho-
rakṣha-virūpākṣha-bileśayāḥ**

*Sri Âdinâtha (Śiva), Matsyendra, Nâtha, Sâbar, Anand,
Bhairava, Chaurangi, Mîna nâtha, Goraksanâtha,
Virupâksa, Bileśaya.*

**6.) manthāno bhairavo yoghī siddhirbudd-
haścha kanthaḍiḥ | koraṃṭakaḥ surānandaḥ
siddhapādaścha charpaṭiḥ**

*Manthâna, Bhairava, Siddhi Buddha, Kanthadi, Karan-
taka, Surânanda, Siddhipâda, Charapati.*

7.) kānerī pūjyapādaścha nitya-nātho nirañjanaḥ | kapālī bindunāthaścha kākachaṇḍīśvarāhvayaḥ

Kânerî, Pûjyapâda, Nityanâtha, Nirañjana, Kapâli, Vindunâtha, Kâka Chandîśwara.

8.) allāmaḥ prabhudevaścha ghoḍā cholī cha ṭimṭiṇiḥ | bhānukī nāradevaścha khaṇḍaḥ kāpālikastathā

Allâma, Prabhudeva, Ghodâ, Cholî, Tintini, Bhânukî Nârdeva, Khanda Kâpâlika, etc.

9.) ityādayo mahāsiddhā haṭha-yogha-prabhā-vataḥ | khaṇḍayitvā kāla-daṇḍaṃ brahmāṇḍe vicharanti te

These Mahâsiddhas (great masters), having conque-red death through the power of Hatha Yoga, roam the universe.

10.) aśeṣha-tāpa-taptānāṃ samāśraya-maṭho haṭhaḥ | aśeṣha-yogha-yuktānāmādhāra-ka-maṭho haṭhaḥ

Hatha is the sanctuary for those suffering every type of pain.

It is the foundation for those practicing every type of Yoga.

11.) haṭha-vidyā paraṃ ghopyā yoghinā siddhimichchatā | bhavedvīryavatī ghuptā nirvīryā tu prakāśitā

A Yogî desirous of success should keep the knowledge of Hatha Yoga secret; for it becomes potent by concealing, and impotent by exposing.

12.) surājye dhārmike deśe subhikṣhe ni-rupadrave | dhanuḥ pramāṇa-paryantaṃ śilāghni-jala-varjite | ekānte maṭhikā-madhye sthātavyaṃ haṭha-yoghinā

The Yogî should practise Hatha Yoga in a small room, situated in a solitary place, being 4 cubits square, and free from stones, fire, water, disturbances of all kinds, and in a country where justice is properly administered, where good people live, and food can be obtained easily and plentifully.

13.) alpa-dvāramarandhra-gharta-vivaraṃ nātyuchcha-nīchāyataṃ samyagh-gho-maya-sāndra-liptamamalaṃ niḥśesa-jantūjjhi-tam | bāhye maṇḍapa-vedi-kūpa-ruchiraṃ prākāra-saṃveṣhṭitaṃ proktaṃ yog-

**ha-maṭhasya lakṣhaṇamidaṃ siddhair-
haṭhābhyāsibhiḥ**

*The room should have a small door, be free from holes,
hollows, neither too high nor too low, well plastered
with cow-dung and free from dirt, filth and insects.
On its outside there should be bowers, raised platform
(chabootrâ), a well, and a compound. These characteristics of a room for Hatha Yogîs have been described by
adepts in the practice of Hatha.*

**14.) aevaṃ vidhe maṭhe sthitvā sar-
va-chintā-vivarjitaḥ I ghurūpadiṣhṭa-mārg-
heṇa yoghameva samabhyaset**

*Having seated in such a room and free from all anxie-
ties, he should practise Yoga, as instructed by his Guru.*

**15.) atyāhāraḥ prayāsaścha prajalpo niy-
amāghrahaḥ I jana-sangghaścha laulyaṃ
cha ṣhaḍbhiryogho vinaśyati**

*Yoga perishes by these six: overeating, overexertion,
talking too much, performing needless austerities, soci-
al-izing, and restlessness.*

16.) utsāhātsāhasāddhairyāttattva-jñānāścha

niśchayāt | jana-sanggha-parityāg-
hātṣhaḍbhiryoghaḥ prasiddhyati

Yoga succeeds by these six: enthusiasm, openness, coura-
ge, knowledge of the truth, determination, and solitude.

17.) atha yama-niyamāḥ ahiṃsā satyamastey-
am brahmacharyaṃ kṣhamā dhṛtiḥ | dayārja-
vaṃ mitāhāraḥ śauchaṃ chaiva yamā daśa

The ten rules of conduct are: ahimsâ (non-injuring),
truth, non-stealing, continence, forgiveness, endurance,
compassion, meekness, sparing diet and cleanliness.

18.) tapaḥ santoṣha āstikyaṃ dānamīśva-
ra-pūjanam | siddhānta-vākya-śravaṇaṃ
hrīmatī cha tapo hutam | niyamā daśa
samproktā yogha-śāstra-viśāradaiḥ

The ten niyamas mentioned by those proficient in the
knowledge of yoga are: Tapa, patience, belief in God,
charity, adoration of God, hearing discourses on the
principles of religion, shame, intellect, Tapa and Yajña.

19.) atha āsanam haṭhasya prathamānggghat-
vādāsanaṃ pūrvamuchyate | kuryāttadāsa-
nam sthairyamāroghyaṃ chānggha-lāghavam

Being the first accessory of Hatha Yoga, âsana is described first. It should be practised for gaining steady posture, health and lightness of body.

20.) vaśiṣṭhādyaiścha munibhirmatsyendrādyaiścha yoghibhiḥ I angghīkṛtānyāsanāni kathyante kānichinmayā

I am going to describe certain âsanas which have been adopted by Munîs like Vasistha and Yogîs like Matsyendra.

21.) jānūrvorantare samyakkṛtvā pāda-tale ubhe I ṝju-kāyaḥ samāsīnaḥ svastikaṃ tat-prachakṣhate

Swastika-âsana.

Having kept both the hands under both the thighs, with the body straight, when one sits calmly in this posture, it is called Swastika.

22.) savye dakṣhiṇa-ghulkaṃ tu pṛṣhṭha-pārśve niyojayet I dakṣhiṇe|api tathā savyam ghomukhaṃ ghomukhākṛtiḥ

Gomukha-âsana.

Placing the right ankle on the left side and the left ankle on the right side, makes Gomukha-âsana, having the appearance of a cow.

23.) ekaṃ pādaṃ tathaikasminvinyasederuṇi sthiram | itarasmiṃstathā choruṃ vīrāsana-mitīritam

Vîrâsana.

One foot is to be placed on the thigh of the opposite side; and so also the other foot on the opposite thigh. This is called Vîrâsana.

24.) ghudaṃ nirudhya ghulphābhyāṃ vyut-krameṇa samāhitaḥ | kūrmāsanaṃ bhavede-taditi yogha-vido viduḥ

Kurmâsana.

Placing the right ankle on the left side of anus, and the left ankle on the right side of it, makes what the Yogîs call Kûrma-âsana.

25.) padmāsanaṃ tu saṃsthāpya jānūrvoran-tare karau | niveśya bhūmau saṃsthāpya vyomasthaṃ kukkuṭāsanam

Kukkuta-âsana.

Taking the posture of Padma-âsana and carrying the hands under the thighs, when the Yogî raises himself above the ground, with his palms resting on the ground, it becomes Kukkuta-âsana.

26.) kukkuṭāsana-bandha-stho dorbhyāṃ sambadya kandharām I bhavedkūrmavaduttāna etaduttāna-kūrmakam

Uttâna Kûrma-âsana.

Having assumed Kukkuta-âsana, when one grasps his neck by crossing his hands behind his head, and lies in this posture with his back touching the ground, it becomes Uttâna Kûrma-âsana, from its appearance like that of a tortoise.

27.) pādāngghuṣhṭhau tu pāṇibhyāṃ ghṛhītvā śravaṇāvadhi I dhanurākarṣhaṇaṃ kuryāddhanur-āsanamuchyate

Dhanura-âsana.

Having caught the toes of the feet with both the hands and carried them to the ears by drawing the body like a bow, it becomes Dhanura âsana.

28+29.) vāmoru-mūlārpita-daksha-pādaṃ
jānorbahirveṣhṭita-vāma-pādam । praghṝhya
tiṣhṭhetparivartitāngghaḥ śrī-matysanāthodi-
tamāsanaṃ syāt

matsyendra-pīṭhaṃ jaṭhara-pradīptiṃ
prachaṇḍa-rughmaṇḍala-khaṇḍanāstram ।
abhyāsataḥ kuṇḍalinī-prabodhaṃ chandra-st-
hiratvaṃ cha dadāti puṃsām

Matsyendrâsana.

*Having placed the right foot at the root of the left thigh,
let the toe be grasped with the right hand passing over
the back, and having placed the left foot on the right
thigh at its root, let it be grasped with the left hand
passing behind the back. This is the âsana, as explained
by Śri Matsyanâtha.*

*It increases appetite and is an instrument for destroy-
ing the group of the most deadly diseases. Its practice
awakens the Kundalinî, stops the nectar shedding from
the moon in people.*

30.) prasārya pādau bhuvi daṇḍa-rūpau dor-
bhyāṃ padāghra-dvitayaṃ ghṝhītvā । jānūpa-
rinyasta-lalāṭa-deśo vasedidaṃ paśchimatā-
namāhuḥ

Paśchima Tâna.

*Having stretched the feet on the ground, like a stick, and
having grasped the toes of both the feet with both the
hands, when one sits with his forehead resting on the
thighs, it is called Paśchima Tâna.*

31.) iti paśchimatānamāsanāghryaṃ pavanaṃ paśchima-vāhinaṃ karoti | udayaṃ jaṭharā-nalasya kuryād udare kārśyamaroghatāṃ cha puṃsām

*This Paśchima Tâna carries the air from the front to the
back part of the body (i.e., to the sushumna). It kindles
gastric fire, reduces obesity and cures all diseases of men.*

32.) dharāmavaṣhṭabhya kara-dvayena tat-kūrpara-sthāpita-nābhi-pārśvaḥ | uchchā-sano daṇḍavadutthitaḥ khe māyūrametatpra-vadanti pīṭham

Mayûra-âsana.

*Place the palms of both the hands on the ground, and
place the navel on both the elbows and balancing thus,
the body should be stretched backward like a stick. This
is called Mayûra-âsana.*

33.) harati sakala-roghānāśu ghulmodarādīn abhibhavati cha doṣhānāsanaṃ śrī-mayūram I bahu kadaśana-bhuktaṃ bhasma kuryā-daśeṣhaṃ janayati jaṭharāghniṃ jārayet-kāla-kūṭam

This Âsana soon destroys all diseases, and removes abdominal disorders, and also those arising from irregularities of phlegm, bile and wind, digests unwholesome food taken in excess, increases appetite and destroys the most deadly poison.

34.) uttānaṃ śabavadbhūmau śayanaṃ tachchavāsanam I śavāsanaṃ śrānti-haraṃ chitta-viśrānti-kārakam

Śava-âsana.

Lying down on the ground, like a corpse, is called Śava-âsana. It removes fatigue and gives rest to the mind.

35.) chaturaśītyāsanāni śivena kathitāni cha I tebhyaśchatuṣhkamādāya sārabhūtaṃ bravī-myaham

Śiva taught 84 âsanas. Of these the first four being essential ones, I am going to explain them here.

**36.) siddhaṃ padmaṃ tathā siṃhaṃ bhadraṃ
veti chatuṣhṭayam । śreṣhṭham tatrāpi cha
sukhe tiṣhṭhetsiddhāsane sadā**

*These four are: The Siddha, Padma, Sinha and Bhadra.
Even of these, the Siddha-âsana, being very comfortable,
one should always practise it.*

**37.) atha siddhāsanam
yoni-sthānakamangghri-mūla-ghaṭitaṃ kṛtvā
dṛḍham vinyaset meṇdhre pādamathaikame-
va hṛdaye kṛtvā hanuṃ susthiram । sthāṇuḥ
saṃyamitendriyo|achala-dṛśā paśyedbh-
ruvorantaraṃ hyetanmokṣha-kapāṭa-bhe-
da-janakaṃ siddhāsanam prochyate**

The Siddhâsana.

*Press firmly the heel of the left foot against the peri-
neum, and the right heel above the male organ. With
the chin pressing on the chest, one should sit calmly,
having restrained the senses, and gaze steadily the space
between the eyebrows. This is called the Siddha Âsana,
the opener of the door of salvation.*

**38.) meṇdhrādupari vinyasya savyaṃ
ghulphaṃ tathopari । ghulphāntaraṃ cha
nikṣhipya siddhāsanamidaṃ bhavet**

This Siddhâsana is performed also by placing the left heel on Medhra (above the male organ), and then placing the right one on it.

39.) etatsiddhāsanaṃ prāhuranye vajrāsanaṃ viduḥ | muktāsanaṃ vadantyeke prāhurg-huptāsanaṃ pare

Some call this Siddhâsana, some Vajrâsana. Others call it Mukta Âsana or Gupta Âsana.

40.) syameṣhviva mitāhāramahiṃsā niya-meṣhviva | mukhyaṃ sarvāsaneṣhvekaṃ siddhāḥ siddhāsanaṃ viduḥ

Just as sparing food is among Yamas, and Ahimsâ among the Niyamas, so is Siddhâsana called by adepts the chief of all the âsanas.

41.) chaturaśīti-pītheshu siddhameva sadābhyaset | dvāsaptati-sahasrānām nādīnām mala-śodhanam

Out of the 84 Âsanas Siddhâsana should always be practised, because it cleanses the impurities of 72,000 nâdîs.

**42.) ātma-dhyāyī mitāhārī yāvaddvādaśa-vat-
saram | sadā siddhāsanābhyāsādyoghī
nishpattimāpnuyāt**

*By contemplating on oneself, by eating sparingly, and
by practising Siddhâsana for 12 years, the Yogî obtains
success.*

**43.) kimanyairbahubhiḥ pīṭhaiḥ siddhe sidd-
hāsane sati | prāṇānile sāvadhāne baddhe
kevala-kumbhake | utpadyate nirāyāsātsvay-
amevonmanī kalā**

*Other postures are of no use, when success has been
achieved in Siddhâsana, and Prâna Vâyû becomes calm
and restrained by Kevala Kumbhaka.*

**44.) tathaikāsminneva drdhe siddhe siddhā-
sane sati | bandha-trayamanāyāsātsvaya-
mevopajāyate**

*Success in one Siddhâsana alone becoming firmly esta-
blished, one gets Unmanî at once, and the three bonds
(Bandhas) are accomplished of themselves.*

**45.) nāsanaṃ siddha-sadṛśaṃ na kumbhaḥ
kevalopamaḥ | na khecharī-samā mudrā na
nāda-sadṛśo layaḥ**

*There is no Âsana like the Siddhâsana and no Kumbha-
ka like the Kevala. There is no mudrâ like the Khechari
and no laya like the Nâda (Anâhata Nâda.)*

**46.) atha padmāsanam
vāmorūpari dakṣiṇaṃ cha charaṇaṃ
saṃsthāpya vāmaṃ tathā dakṣhorūpa-
ri paśchimena vidhinā dhṛtvā karābhyāṃ
dṛḍham | angghuṣhṭhau hṛdaye nidhāya
chibukaṃnāsāghramālokayet etadvyād-
hi-vināśa-kāri yamināṃ padmāsanaṃ prochyate**

The Padmâsana.

*Place the right foot on the left thigh and the left foot on
the right thigh, and grasp the toes with the hands crossed
over the back. Press the chin against the chest and gaze
on the tip of the nose. This is called the Padmâsana, the
destroyer of the diseases of the Yamîs.*

**47.) uttānau charaṇau kṛtvā ūru-saṃsthau
prayatnataḥ | ūru-madhye tathottānau pāṇī
kṛtvā tato dṛśau**

*Place the feet on the thighs, with the soles upwards, and
place the hands on the thighs, with the palms upwards.*

**48.) nāsāghre vinyasedrājad-anta-mūle tu
jihvayā I uttambhya chibukaṃ vakṣhasyutt-
hāpy pavanaṃ śanaiḥ**

*Gaze on the tip of the nose, keeping the tongue pressed
against the root of the teeth of the upper jaw, and the
chin against the chest, and raise the air up slowly, i.e.,
pull the apâna-vâyû gently upwards.*

**49.) idaṃ padmāsanaṃ proktaṃ sarva-vyād-
hi-vināśanam I durlabhaṃ yena kenāpi
dhīmatā labhyate bhuvi**

*This is called the Padmâsana, the destroyer of all dise-
ases. It is difficult of attainment by everybody, but can
be learnt by intelligent people in this world.*

**50.) kṛtvā sampuṭitau karau dṛḍhataraṃ badd-
hvā tu padmamāsanaṃ ghāḍhaṃ vakṣhasi
sannidhāya chibukaṃ dhyāyaṃścha tach-
chetasi I vāraṃ vāramapānamūrdhvamanilaṃ
protsārayanpūritaṃ nyañchanprāṇamupaiti
bodhamatulaṃ śakti-prabhāvānnaraḥ**

*Having kept both the hands together in the lap, perfor-
ming the Padmâsana firmly, keeping the chin Fixed to
the chest and contemplating on Him in the mind, by
drawing the apâna-vâyû up (performing Mûla Bandha)*

and pushing down the air after inhaling it, joining thus the prâna and apâna in the navel, one gets the highest intelligence by awakening the śakti (kundalinî) thus.

NB.—When Apâna Vâyû is drawn gently up and after filling in the lungs with the air from outside, the prâna is forced down by and by so as to join both of them in the navel, they both enter then the Kundalinî and, reaching the Brahma randhra (the great hole), they make the mind calm. Then the mind can contemplate on the nature of the âtmana and can enjoy the highest bliss.

51.) padmāsane sthito yoghī nāḍī-dvāreṇa pūritam mārutaṃ dhārayedyastu sa mukto nātra saṃśayaḥ

The Yogî who, sitting with Padmâsana, can control breathing, there is no doubt, is free from bondage.

52.) atha siṃhāsanam
ghulphau cha vṛṣhaṇasyādhaḥ sīvantyāḥ pārśvayoḥ kṣhipet I dakṣhiṇe savya-ghulpham tu dakṣha- ghulpham tu savyake

The Simhâsana.

Press the heels on both sides of the seam of Perineum, in

*such a way that the left heel touches the right side and
the right heel touches the left side of it.*

53.) hastau tu jānvoḥ saṃsthāpya svāngg-hulīḥ sam-prasārya cha | vyātta-vakto nirīkṣ-heta nāsāgh-raṃ susamāhitaḥ

*Place the hands on the thighs, with stretched fingers,
and keeping the mouth open and the mind collected,
gaze on the tip of the nose.*

54.) siṃhāsanaṃ bhavedetatpūjitaṃ yog-hi-pungghavaiḥ | bandha-tritaya-sandhānaṃ kurute chāsanottamam

*This is Simhâsana, held sacred by the best of Yogîs. This
excellent Âsana effects the completion of the three Bandhas (The Mûlabandha, Kantha or Jâlandhar Bandha
and Uddiyâna Bandha).*

55+56.) atha bhadrāsanam ghulphau cha vṛṣhaṇasyādhaḥ sīvantyāḥ pārśvayoḥ kṣhipte | savya-ghulphaṃ tathā savye dakṣha-ghulphaṃ tu dakṣhiṇe

pārśva-pādau cha pāṇibhyāṃ dṛḍhaṃ baddh-vā suniśchalam | bhadrāsanaṃ bhavedetats-arva-vyādhi-vināśanam | ghorakṣhāsanami-tyāhuridaṃ vai siddha-yoghinaḥ

The Bhadrâsana.

*Place the heels on either side of the seam of the Peri-
neum, keeping the left heel on the left side and the right
one on the right side, hold the feet firmly joined to one
another with both the hands. This Bhadrâsana is the
destroyer of all the diseases.*

57.) evamāsana-bandheṣhu yoghīndro vig-hata-śramaḥ । abhyasennāḍikā-śuddhiṃ mudrādi-pavanī-kriyām

*The expert Yogîs call this Gorakśa âsana. By sitting with
this âsana, the Yogî gets rid of fatigue.*

58.) āsanaṃ kumbhakam chitraṃ mudrākhy-am karaṇam tathā । atha nādānusandhāna-mabhyāsānukramo haṭhe

*The Nâdis should be cleansed of their impurities by
performing the mudrâs, etc. (which are the practices
relating to the air). Âsanas, Kumbhakas and various
curious mûdrâs.*

59.) brahmachārī mitāhārī tyāghī yog-ha-parāyaṇaḥ । abdādūrdhvaṃ bhavedsidd-ho nātra kāryā vichāraṇā

*By regular and close attention to Nâda (anâhata nâda)
in Hatha Yoga, a Brahmachari, sparing in diet, unat-
tached to objects of enjoyment, and devoted to Yoga,
gains success, no doubt, within a year.*

60.) susnighdha-madhurāhāraścha-
turthāṃśa-vivarjitaḥ ǀ bhujyate śi-
va-samprītyai mitāhāraḥ sa uchyate

*Abstemious feeding is that in which ¾ of hunger is sa-
tisfied with food, well cooked with ghee and sweets, and
eaten with the offering of it to Śiva.*

61.) kaṭvāmla-tīkṣhṇa-lavaṇoṣhṇa-harīta-śāka-
sauvīra-taila-tila-sarṣhapa-madya-matsyān
ǀ ājādi-māṃsa-dadhi-takra-kulatthakola-
piṇyāka-hingghu-laśunādyamapathyamāhuḥ

Foods injurious to a Yogî.

*Bitter, sour, saltish, hot, green vegetables, fermented,
oily, mixed with til seed, rape seed, intoxicating liquors,
fish, meat, curds, chhaasa pulses, plums, oil-cake, asafo-
etida (hînga), garlic, onion, etc. should not be eaten.*

62.) sbhojanamahitaṃ vidyātpuna-
rasyoṣhṇī-kṛtaṃ rūkṣham ǀ atilavaṇamam-
la-yuktaṃ kadaśana-śākotkaṃ varjyam

Food heated again, dry, having too much salt, sour, minor grains, and vegetables that cause burning sensation, should not be eaten, Fire, women, travelling, etc., should be avoided.

63.) vahni-strī-pathi-sevānāmādau varja-namācharet

As said by Goraksa, one should keep aloof from the society of the evil-minded, fire, women, travelling, early morning bath, fasting, and all kinds of bodily exertion.

64.) tathā hi ghoraksha-vachanam varjayed-durjana-prāntam vahni-strī-pathi-sevanam I prātaḥ-snānopavāsādi kāya-kleśa-vidhim tathā

Wheat, rice, barley, shâstik (a kind of rice), good corns, milk, ghee, sugar, butter, sugarcandy, honey, dried ginger, Parwal (a vegetable) the five vegetables, moong, pure water, these are very beneficial to those who practise Yoga.

65.) hodhūma-śāli-yava-ṣhāṣhṭika-śobhanān-nam kṣhīrājya-khaṇḍa-navanīta-sidd-hā-madhūni I śuṇṭhī-paṭola-kaphalādi-ka-pañcha-śākam mudghādi-divyamudakam cha yamīndra-pathyam

*A Yogî should eat tonics (things giving strength), well
sweetened, greasy (made with ghee), milk, butter, etc.,
which may increase humors of the body, according to his
desire.*

66.) puṣhṭaṃ sumadhuraṃ snighdhaṃ ghavy-aṃ dhātu-praposhaṇam I manobhilaṣhitaṃ yoghyaṃ yoghī bhojanamācharet

*Whether young, old or too old, sick or lean, one who
discards laziness, gets success if he practises Yoga.*

67.) yuvo vṛddho|ativṛddho vā vyādhito dur-balo|api vā I abhyāsātsiddhimāpnoti sar-va-yogheṣhvatandritaḥ

*Success comes to him who is engaged in the practice.
How can one get success without practice; for by merely
reading books on Yoga, one can never get success.*

68.) kriyā-yuktasya siddhiḥ syādakriyasya kathaṃ bhavet I na śāstra-pāṭha-mātreṇa yogha-siddhiḥ prajāyate

*Success cannot be attained by adopting a particular
dress (Vesa). It cannot be gained by telling tales. Practice
alone is the means to success. This is true, there is no
doubt.*

69+70.) na veṣha-dhāraṇaṃ siddheḥ kāraṇaṃ na cha tat-kathā | kriyaiva kāraṇaṃ siddheḥ satyametanna saṃśayaḥ

pīṭhāni kumbhakāśchitrā divyāni karaṇāni cha | sarvāṇyapi haṭhābhyāse rāja-yog-ha-phalāvadhi

Âsanas (postures), various Kumbhakas, and other divine means, all should be practised in the practice of Hatha Yoga, till the fruit—Râja Yoga—is obtained.

iti haṭha-pradīpikāyāṃ prathamopadeśaḥ

End of chapter 1st, on the method of forming the Âsa-
nas.

Chapter 2

Pranayamas

Dvitīyopadeśah

**1.) athāsane dṛdhe yoghī vaśī hita-mitāśanaḥ
| ghurūpadiṣhṭa-mārgheṇa prāṇāyāmānsam-
abhyaset**

*Posture becoming established, a Yogî, master of himself,
eating salutary and moderate food, should practise
Prânâyâma, as instructed by his guru.*

**2.) chale vāte chalaṃ chittaṃ niśchale
niśchalaṃ bhavet II yoghī sthāṇutvamāpnoti
tato vāyuṃ nirodhayet**

*Respiration being disturbed, the mind becomes distur-
bed. By restraining respiration, the Yogî gets steadiness
of mind.*

**3.) yāvadvāyuḥ sthito dehe tāvajjīvanamuchy-
ate I maraṇaṃ tasya niṣhkrāntistato vāyuṃ
nirodhayet**

*So long as the (breathing) air stays in the body, it is
called life. Death consists in the passing out of the
(breathing) air. It is, therefore, necessary to restrain the
breath.*

**4.) malākalāsu nāḍīṣhu māruto naiva mad-
hyaghaḥ | kathaṃ syādunmanībhāvaḥ
kārya-siddhiḥ kathaṃ bhavet**

*The breath does not pass through the middle channel
(susumnâ), owing to the impurities of the nâdîs. How
can then success be attained, and how can there be the
unmanî avasthâ.*

**5.) śuddhameti yadā sarvaṃ nāḍī-chakraṃ
malākulam | tadaiva jāyate yoghī
prāṇa-saṃghrahaṇe kṣhamaḥ**

*When the whole system of nâdîs which is full of impuri-
ties, is cleaned, then the Yogî becomes able to control the
Prâna.*

**6.) prāṇāyāmaṃ tataḥ kuryānnityaṃ sātt-
vikayā dhiyā | yathā suṣhumṇā-nāḍīsthā
malāḥ śuddhiṃ prayānti cha**

*Therefore, Prânâyâma should be performed daily with
sâtwika buddhi (intellect free from raja and tama or
activity and sloth), in order to drive out the impurities of
the susumnâ.*

7+8.) baddha-padmāsano yoghī prāṇaṃ

chandreṇa pūrayet | dhārayitvā yathā-śakti bhūyaḥ sūryeṇa rechayet

prāṇaṃ sūryeṇa chākṛṣhya pūrayedudaraṃ śanaiḥ | vidhivatkumbhakaṃ kṛtvā punaśchandreṇa rechayet

Method of performing Prânâyâma.

Sitting in the Padmâsana posture the Yogî should fill in the air through the left nostril (closing the right one); and, keeping it confined according to one's ability, it should be expelled slowly through the sûrya (right nostril). Then, drawing in the air through the sûrya (right nostril) slowly, the belly should be filled, and after performing Kumbhaka as before, it should be expelled slowly through the chandra (left nostril).

9.) yena tyajettena pītvā dhārayedatirodhataḥ | rechayechcha tato|anyena śanaireva na veghataḥ

Inhaling thus through the one, through which it was expelled, and having restrained it there, till possible, it should be exhaled through the other, slowly and not forcibly.

10.) prāṇaṃ chediḍayā pibenniyamitaṃ

bhūyo I anyathā rechayet pītvā pingghalayā
samīraṇamatho baddhvā tyajedvāmayā I
sūrya-chandramasoranena vidhinābhyāsaṃ
sadā tanvatāṃ śuddhā nāḍi-ghaṇā bhavanti
yamināṃ māsa-trayādūrdhvataḥ

*If the air be inhaled through the left nostril, it should be
expelled again through the other, and filling it through
the right nostril, confining it there, it should be expelled through the left nostril. By practising in this way,
through the right and the left nostrils alternately, the
whole of the collection of the nâdîs of the yamîs (prac-
tisers) becomes clean, i.e., free from impurities, after 3
months and over.*

11.) prātarmadhyandine sāyamardha-rātre cha kumbhakān I śanairaśīti-paryantaṃ chatur-vāraṃ samabhyaset

*Kumbhakas should be performed gradually 4 times
during day and night, i.e., (morning, noon, evening and
midnight), till the number of Kumbhakas for one time is
80 and for day and night together it is 320.*

12.) kanīyasi bhavedsveda kampo bhavati madhyame I uttame sthānamāpnoti tato vāy-uṃ nibandhayet

In the beginning there is perspiration, in the middle stage there is quivering, and in the last or the 3rd stage one obtains steadiness; and then the breath should be made steady or motionless.

13.) jalena śrama-jātena ghātra-marda-namācharet I dṛḍhatā laghutā chaiva tena ghātrasya jāyate

The perspiration exuding from exertion of practice should be rubbed into the body (and not wiped), as by so doing the body becomes strong.

14.) abhyāsa-kāle prathame śastaṃ kṣhīrājya-bhojanam I tato|abhyāse dṛḍhībhū-te na tādṛng-niyama-ghrahaḥ

During the first stage of practice the food consisting of milk and ghee is wholesome. When the practice becomes established, no such restriction is necessary.

15.) yathā siṃho ghajo vyāghro bhavedvaśy-aḥ śanaiḥ śanaiḥ I tathaiva sevito vāyurany-athā hanti sādhakam

Just as lions, elephants and tigers are controlled by and by, so the breath is controlled by slow degrees, otherwise (i.e., by being hasty or using too much force) it kills the practiser himself.

16.) prāṇāyāmena yuktena sarva-rog-ha-kṣhayo bhavet I ayuktābhyāsa-yoghena sarva-rogha-samudghamaḥ

When Prânayama, etc., are performed properly, they eradicate all diseases; but an improper practice generates diseases.

17.) hikkā śvāsaścha kāsaścha śi-raḥ-karṇākṣhi-vedanāḥ I bhavanti vividhāḥ roghāḥ pavanasya prakopataḥ

Hiccough, asthma, cough, pain in the head, the ears, and the eyes; these and other various kinds of diseases are generated by the disturbance of the breath.

18.) yuktaṃ yuktaṃ tyajedvāyuṃ yuktaṃ yuktaṃ cha pūrayet I yuktaṃ yuktaṃ cha badhnīyādevaṃ siddhimavāpnuyāt

The air should be expelled with proper tact and should be filled in skilfully; and when it has been kept confined properly it brings success.

NB.—The above caution is necessary to warn the aspi-

*rants against omitting any instruction; and, in their zeal
to gain success or siddhis early, to begin the practice,
either by using too much force in filling in, confining
and expelling the air, or by omitting any instructions,
it may cause unnecessary pressure on their ears, eyes,
&c,, and cause pain. Every word in the instructions is
full of meaning and is necessarily used in the slokas, and
should be followed very carefully and with due attention. Thus there will be nothing to fear whatsoever. We
are inhaling and exhaling the air throughout our lives
without any sort of danger, and Prânayama being only
a regular form of it, there should be no cause to fear.*

19.) yadā tu nāḍī-śuddhiḥ syāttathā chihnāni bāhyataḥ I kāyasya kṛśatā kāntistadā jāyate niśchitam

*When the nâdîs become free from impurities, and there
appear the outward signs of success, such as lean body
and glowing colour, then one should feel certain of
success.*

20.) yatheshṭaṃ dhāraṇaṃ vāyoranalasya pradīpanam I nādābhivyaktirāroghyaṃ jāya-te nāḍi-śodhanāt

By removing the impurities, the air can be restrained,

*according to one's wish and the appetite is increased,
the divine sound is awakened, and the body becomes
healthy.*

21.) meda-śleṣhmādhikaḥ pūrvaṃ ṣhaṭ-karmāṇi samācharet | anyastu nācharettāni doṣhāṇāṃ samabhāvataḥ

*If there be excess of fat or phlegm in the body, the six
kinds of kriyâs (duties) should be performed first. But
others, not suffering from the excess of these, should not
perform them.*

22.) dhautirbastistathā netistrāṭakaṃ nau-likaṃ tathā | kapāla-bhātiśchaitāni ṣhaṭ-karmāṇi prachakṣhate

*The six kinds of duties are: Dhauti, Basti, Neti, Trâtaka,
Nauti and Kapâla Bhâti. These are called the six actions.*

23.) karma ṣhaṭkamidaṃ ghopyaṃ ghaṭa-śod-hana-kārakam | vichitra-ghuṇa-sandhāya pūjyate yoghi-pungghavaiḥ

*These six kinds of actions which cleanse the body should
be kept secret. They produce extraordinary attributes
and are performed with earnestness by the best of Yogîs.*

**24.) tatra dhautiḥ
chatur-angghula-vistāraṃ has-
ta-pañcha-daśāyatam | ghurūpadiṣhṭa-mārg-
heṇa siktaṃ vastraṃ śanairghraset | punaḥ
pratyāharechchaitaduditaṃ dhauti-karma tat**

The Dhauti.

*A strip of cloth, about 3 inches wide and 15 cubits long,
is pushed in (swallowed), when moist with warm water,
through the passage shown by the guru, and is taken out
again. This is called Dhauti Karma.*

*NB.—The strip should be moistened with a little warm
water, and the end should be held with the teeth. It is
swallowed slowly, little by little; thus, first day 1 cubit,
2nd day 2 cubits, 3rd day 3 cubits, and so on. After
swallowing it the stomach should be given a good, round
motion from left to right, and then it should be taken
out slowly and gently.*

**25.) kāsa-śvāsa-plīha-kuṣhṭhaṃ kapharog-
hāścha vimśatiḥ | dhauti-karma-prabhāveṇa
prayāntyeva na saṃśayaḥ**

*There is no doubt, that cough, asthma, enlargement
of the spleen, leprosy, and 20 kinds of diseases born of
phlegm, disappear by the practice of Dhauti Karma.*

26.) atha bastiḥ
nābhi-daghna-jale pāyau nyasta-nālotkaṭās-
anaḥ | ādhārākuñchanaṃ kuryātkṣhālanaṃ
basti-karma tat

The Basti.

*Squatting in navel-deep water, and introducing a six
inches long, smooth piece of ½ an inch diameter pipe,
open at both ends, half inside the anus; it (anus) should
he drawn up (contracted) and then expelled. This
washing is called the Basti Karma.*

27.) ghulma-plīhodaraṃ chāpi vāta-pitta-kap-
hodbhavāḥ | basti-karma-prabhāveṇa kṣhīy-
ante sakalāmayāḥ

*By practising this Basti Karma, colic, enlarged spleen,
and dropsy, arising from the disorders of Vâta (air),
pitta (bile) and kapha (phlegm), are all cured.*

28.) dhāntvadriyāntaḥ-karaṇa-prasādaṃ
dadhāchcha kāntiṃ dahana-pradīptam |
aśeṣha-doṣhopachayaṃ nihanyād abhyasy-
amānaṃ jala-basti-karma

*By practising Basti with water, the Dhâtâs, the Indriyas
and the mind become calm. It gives glow and tone to*

*the body and increases the appetite. All the disorders
disappear.*

29.) atha netiḥ
**sūtraṃ vitasti-susnighdhaṃ nāsānāle pra-
veśayet | mukhānnirghamayechchaiṣhā
netiḥ siddhairnighadyate**

The Neti.

*A cord made of threads and about six inches long,
should be passed through the passage of the nose and
the end taken out in the mouth. This is called by adepts
the Neti Karma.*

30.) kapāla-śodhinī chaiva divya-dṛṣhṭi-
**pradāyinī | jatrūrdhva-jāta-roghaughaṃ
netirāśu nihanti cha**

*The Neti is the cleaner of the brain and giver of divine
sight. It soon destroys all the diseases of the cervical and
scapular regions.*

31.) atha trāṭakam
**nirīkṣhenniśchala-dṛśā sūkṣhma-lakṣhyaṃ
samāhitaḥ | aśru-sampāta-paryantamāchāry-
aistrāṭakaṃ smṛtam**

The Trâtaka.

*Being calm, one should gaze steadily at a small mark,
till eyes are filled with tears. This is called Trataka by
âchâryas.*

32.) mochanaṃ netra-roghāṇāṃ tandādrīṇāṃ kapāṭakam I yatnatastrāṭakaṃ ghopyaṃ yathā hāṭaka-peṭakam

*Trâtaka destroys the eye diseases and removes sloth,
etc. It should be kept secret very carefully, like a box of
jewellery.*

33.) atha nauliḥ amandāvarta-veghena tundaṃ savyāpasavya-taḥ I natāṃso bhrāmayedeṣhā nauliḥ sidd-haiḥ praśasyate

The Nauli.

*Sitting on the toes with heels raised above the ground,
and the palms resting on the ground, and in this bent
posture the belly is moved forcibly from left to right just,
as in vomiting. This is called by adepts the Nauli Karma.*

**34.) mandāghni-sandīpana-pāchanādi-sand-
hāpikānanda-karī sadaiva | aśeṣa-doṣha-
maya-śoṣhaṇī cha haṭha-kriyā mauliriyaṃ
cha nauliḥ**

*It removes dyspepsia, increases appetite and digestion,
and is like the goddess of creation, and causes happiness.
It dries up all the disorders. This Nauli is an excellent
exercise in Hatha Yoga.*

**35.) atha kapālabhātiḥ
bhastrāvalloha-kārasya recha-pūrau sasam-
bhramau | kapālabhātirvikhyātā kapha-
doṣha-viśoṣhaṇī**

The Kapâla Bhâti.

*When inhalation and exhalation are performed very
quickly, like a pair of bellows of a blacksmith, it dries
up all the disorders from the excess of phlegm, and is
known as Kapâla Bhâti.*

**36.) ṣhaṭ-karma-nirghata-sthaulya-kap-
ha-doṣha-malādikaḥ | prāṇāyāmaṃ tataḥ
kuryādanāyāsena siddhyati**

When Prânâyâma is performed after getting rid of

*obesity born of the defects phlegm, by the performance
of the six duties, it easily brings success.*

37.) prāṇāyāmaireva sarve praśuṣhyanti malā iti I āchāryāṇāṃ tu keṣhāṃchidanyatkarma na saṃmatam

*Some âchâryâs (teachers) do not advocate any other
practice, being of opinion that all the impurities are
dried up by the practice of Prânâyâma.*

38.) atha ghaja-karaṇī udara-ghata-padārthamudvamanti pavana-mapānamudīrya kaṇṭha-nāle I krama-pa-richaya-vaśya-nāḍi-chakrā ghaja-karaṇīti nighadyate haṭhajñaiḥ

Gaja Karani.

*By carrying the Apâna Vâyû up to the throat, the food,
etc., in the stomach are vomited. By degrees, the system
of Nâdîs (Śankhinî) becomes known. This is called in
Hatha as Gaja Karani.*

39.) brahmādayo|api tridaśāḥ pavanābhyā-sa-tatparāḥ I abhūvannantaka-bhyāttasmāt-pavanamabhyaset

*Brahmâ, and other Devas were always engaged in
the exercise of Prânâyâma, and, by means of it, got
rid of the fear of death. Therefore, one should practise
prânâyâma regularly.*

40.) yāvadbaddho marud-deśe yāvachchit-tam nirākulam I yāvaddṛṣhṭirbhruvormadhye tāvatkāla-bhayaṃ kutaḥ

*So long as the breath is restrained in the body, so long as
the mind is undisturbed, and so long as the gaze is fixed
between the eyebrows, there is no fear from Death.*

41.) vidhivatprāṇa-saṃyāmairnāḍī-chakre viśodhite I suṣhumṇā-vadanaṃ bhittvā suk-hādviśati mārutaḥ

*When the system of Nâdis becomes clear of the impu-
rities by properly controlling the prâna, then the air,
piercing the entrance of the Suśumnâ, enters it easily.*

42.) atha manonmanī marute madhya-saṃchāre manaḥ-sthairy-am prajāyate I yo manaḥ-susthirī-bhāvaḥ saivāvasthā manonmanī

Manomanî.

Steadiness of mind comes when the air moves Freely in the middle. That is the manonmanî condition, which is attained when the mind becomes calm.

43.) tat-siddhaye vidhānajñāśchitrānkurvanti kumbhakān I vichitra kumbhakābhyāsād- vichitrāṃ siddhimāpnuyāt

To accomplish it, various Kumbhakas are performed by those who are expert in the methods; for, by the practice of different Kumbhakas, wonderful success is attained.

44.) atha kumbhaka-bhedāḥ sūrya-bhedanamujjāyī sītkārī śītalī tathā I bhastrikā bhrāmarī mūrchchā plāvinīty- aṣhṭa-kumbhakāḥ

Different hinds of Kumbhakas. Kumbhakas are of eight kinds, viz., Sûrya Bhedan, Ujjâyî, Sîtkarî, Sîtali, Bhas- trikâ, Bhrâmarî, Mûrchhâ, and Plâvinî.

45.) pūrakānte tu kartavyo bandho jāland- harābhidhaḥ I kumbhakānte rechakādau kartavyastūḍḍiyānakaḥ

*At the end of Pûraka, Jâlandhara Bandha should be
performed, and at the end of Kumbhaka, and at the
beginning of Rechaka, Uddiyâna Bandha should be
performed.*

NB.—Pûraka is filling in of the air from outside.

*Kumbhaka is the keeping the air confined inside. Recha-
ka is expelling the confined air. The instructions for
Puraka, Kumbhaka and Rechaka will be found at their
proper place and should he carefully followed.*

46.) adhastātkuñchanenāśu kaṇṭha-sang-kochane kṛte I madhye paśchima-tānena syātprāṇo brahma-nāḍighaḥ

*By drawing up from below (Mûla Bandha) and con-
tracting the throat (Jâlandhara Bandha) and by pulling
back the middle of the front portion of the body (i.e.,
belly), the Prâna goes to the Brahma Nâdî (Susumnâ).*

*The middle hole, through the vertebral column, through
which the spinal cord passes, is called the Susumnâ Nâdî
of the Yogîs. The two other sympathetic cords, one on
each aide of the spinal cord, are called the Idâ and the
Pingalâ Nâdîs. These will be described later on.*

**47.) āpānamūrdhvamutthāpya prāṇaṃ
kaṇṭhādadho nayet I yoghī jarā-vimuktaḥ
sanṣhoḍaśābda-vayā bhavet**

By pulling up the Apâna Vâyu and by forcing the Prâna Vâyu down the throat, the Yogî, liberated from old age, becomes young, as it were 16 years old.

Note.

The seat of the Prâna is the heart; of the Apâna anus; of the Samâna the region about the navel; of the Udâna the throat; while the Vyâna moves throughout the body.

**48.) atha sūrya-bhedanam
āsane sukhade yoghī baddhvā chaivāsanaṃ
tataḥ I dakṣha-nāḍyā samākṛṣhya bahiḥst-
haṃ pavanaṃ śanaiḥ**

Sûrya Bhedana.

Taking any comfortable posture and performing the âsana, the Yogî should draw in the air slowly, through the right nostril.

**49.) ākeśādānakhāghrāchcha nirodhāvad-
hi kumbhayet I tataḥ śanaiḥ savya-nāḍyā
rechayetpavanaṃ śanaiḥ**

Then it should be confined within, so that it fills from the nails to the tips of the hair, and then let out through the left nostril slowly.

Note. This is to be done alternately with both the nostrils, drawing in through the one, expelling through the other, and vice versa.

50.) kapāla-śodhanaṃ vāta-doṣha-ghnaṃ kṛmi-doṣha-hṛt l punaḥ punaridaṃ kāryaṃ sūrya-bhedanamuttamam

This excellent Sûrya Bhedana cleanses the forehead (frontal sinuses), destroys the disorders of Vâta, and removes the worms, and, therefore, it should be performed again and again.

Note.

Translation: I am going to describe the procedure of the practice of Yoga, in order that Yogîs may succeed. A wise man should leave his bed in the Usâ Kâla (i.e. at the peep of dawn or 4 o'clock) in the morning. 1.

Remembering his guru over his head, and his desired deity in his heart, after answering the calls of nature, and cleaning his mouth, he should apply Bhasma (ashes). 2.

*In a clean spot, clean room and charming ground, he
should spread a soft âsana (cloth for sitting on). Having
seated on it and remembering, in his mind his guru and
his God. 3.*

*Having extolled the place and the time and taking up
the vow thus: 'To day by the grace of God, I will perform
Prânâyâmas with âsanas for gaining samâdhi (trance)
and its fruits.' He should salute the infinite Deva, Lord of
the Nâgas, to ensure success in the âsanas (postures). 4.*

*Salutation to the Lord of the Nâgas, who is adorned
with thousands of heads, set with brilliant jewels
(manis), and who has sustained the whole universe, no-
urishes it, and is infinite. After this he should begin his
exercise of âsanas and when fatigued, he should practise
Śava âsana. Should there be no fatigue, he should not
practise it. 5.*

*Before Kumbhaka, he should perform Viparîta Karnî
mudrâ, in order that he may be able to perform Jâlandhar bandha comfortably. 6.*

*Sipping a little water, he should begin the exercise of
Prânâyâma, after saluting Yogindras, as described in the
Karma Parana, in the words of Śiva. 7.*

Such as "Saluting Yogindras and their disciples and gurû

Vinâyaka, the Yogî should unite with me with composed mind." 8.

While practising, he should sit with Siddhâsana, and having performed bandha and Kumbhaka, should begin with 10 Prânâyâmas the first day, and go on increasing 5 daily. 9.

With composed mind 80 Kumbhakas should be performed at a time; beginning first with the chandra (the left nostril) and then sûrya (the right nostril). 10.

This has been spoken of by wise men as Aouloma and Viloma. Having practised Sûrya Bhedan, with Bandhas, the wise rust) should practise Ujjâyî and then Sîtkârî Sîtalî, and Bhastrikâ, he may practice others or not. 11-12.

He should practise mudrâs properly, as instructed by his guru. Then sitting with Padmâsana, he should hear anâhata nâda attentively. 13.

He should resign the fruits of all his practice reverently to God, and, on rising on the completion of the practice, a warm bath should be taken. 14.

The bath should bring all the daily duties briefly to an end. At noon also a little rest should be taken at the end of the exercise, and then food should be taken. 15.

Yogîs should always take wholesome food and never anything unwholesome. After dinner he should eat Ilâchî or lavanga. 16.

Some like camphor, and betel leaf. To the Yogîs, practising Prânâyâma, betel leaf without powders, i, e., lime, nuts and kâtha, is beneficial. 17.

After taking food he should read books treating of salvation, or hear Purânas and repeat the name of God. 18. In the evening the exercise should be begun after finishing sandyhâ, as before, beginning the practice 3 ghatikâ or one hour before the sun sets. 19.

Evening sandhyâ should always be performed after practice, and Hatha Yoga should be practised at midnight. 20.

Viparîta Karni is to be practised in the evening and at midnight, and not just after eating, as it does no good at this time. 21.

51.) atha ujjāyī
mukhaṃ saṃyamya nāḍībhyāmākṛṣhya pava-
nam śanaiḥ । yathā laghati kaṇṭhāttu hṛday-
āvadhi sa-svanam

Ujjâyî.

Having closed the opening of the Nâdî (Larynx), the air should be drawn in such a way that it goes touching from the throat to the chest, and making noise while passing.

52.) pūrvavatkumbhayetprāṇaṃ rechayediḍayā tathā I śleṣhma-doṣha-haraṃ kaṇṭhe dehānala-vivardhanam

It should be restrained, as before, and then let out through Idâ (the left nostril). This removes ślesmâ (phlegm) in the throat and increases the appetite.

53.) nāḍī-jalodarādhātu-ghata-doṣha-vināśanam I ghachchatā tiṣhṭhatā kāryamujjāyyākhyaṃ tu kumbhakam

It destroys the defects of the nâdîs, dropsy and disorders of Dhâtu (humours). Ujjâyî should be performed in all conditions of life, even while walking or sitting.

54.) atha sītkārī
sītkāṃ kuryāttathā vaktre ghrāṇenaiva vijṛmbhikām I evamabhyāsa-yoghena kāma-devo dvitīyakaḥ

Sîtkârî.

Sîtkârî is performed by drawing in the air through the mouth, keeping the tongue between the lips. The air thus drawn in should not be expelled through the mouth. By practising in this way, one becomes next to the God of Love in beauty.

55.) yoghinī chakra-sammānyaḥ sṛṣhṭi-samhāra-kārakaḥ I na kṣhudhā na tṛṣhā nidrā naivālasyaṃ prajāyate

He is regarded adorable by the Yoginîs and becomes the destroyer of the cycle of creation, He is not afflicted with hunger, thirst, sleep or lassitude.

56.) bhavetsattvaṃ cha dehasya sarvopadra-va-varjitaḥ I anena vidhinā satyaṃ yoghīnd-ro bhūmi-maṇḍale

The Satwa of his body becomes free from all the distur-bances. In truth, he becomes the lord of the Yogîs in this world.

57.) atha śītalī
jihvayā vāyumākṛṣhya pūrvavatkumbha-sād-hanam I śanakairghrāṇa-randhrābhyāṃ rechayetpavanaṃ sudhīḥ

Sîtalî.

As in the above (Sîtkári), the tongue to be protruded a little out of the lips, when the air is drawn in. It is kept confined, as before, and then expelled slowly through the nostrils.

58.) ghulma-plīhādikānroghānjvaraṃ pittaṃ kṣhudhāṃ tṛṣhām I viṣhāṇi śītalī nāma kumbhikeyaṃ nihanti hi

This Sîtalî kumbhikâ cures colic, (enlarged) spleen, fever, disorders of bile, hunger, thirst, and counteracts poisons.

59.) atha bhastrikā
ūrvorupari saṃsthāpya śubhe pāda-tale ubhe I padmāsanaṃ bhavedetatsarva-pā-pa-praṇāśanam

The Bhastrikâ.

The Padma Âsana consists in crossing the feet and placing them on both the thighs; it is the destroyer of all sins.

60.) samyakpadmāsanaṃ baddhvā
sama-ghrīvodaraḥ sudhīḥ I mukhaṃ samya-mya yatnena prāṇaṃ ghrāṇena rechayet

*Binding the Padma-Âsana and keeping the body
straight, closing the mouth carefully, let the air be expelled through the nose.*

61.) yathā laghati hṛt-kaṇṭhe kapālāvad-
hi sa-svanam ǀ veghena pūrayechchāpi
hṛt-padmāvadhi mārutam

*It should be filled up to the lotus of the heart, by drawing
it in with force, making noise and touching the throat,
the chest and the head.*

62.) punarvirechayettadvatpūrayechcha
punaḥ punaḥ ǀ yathaiva lohakāreṇa bhastrā
veghena chālyate

*It should he expelled again and filled again and again
as before, just as a pair of bellows of the blacksmith is
worked.*

63.) tathaiva sva-śarīra-sthaṃ chālayetpava-
naṃ dhiyā ǀ yadā śramo bhaveddehe tadā
sūryeṇa pūrayet

*In the same way, the air of the body should be moved
intelligently, filling it through Sûrya when fatigue is
experienced.*

64.) yathodaraṃ bhavetpūrṇamanilena tathā laghu | dhārayennāsikāṃ madhyā-tar-janībhyāṃ vinā dṛḍham

The air should be drawn in through the right nostril by pressing the thumb against the left side of the nose, so as to close the left nostril; and when filled to the full, it should be closed with the fourth finger (the one next to the little finger) and kept confined.

65.) vidhivatkumbhakaṃ kṛtvā rechayediḍay-ānilam | vāta-pitta-śleṣhma-haraṃ śarīrāgh-ni-vivardhanam

Having confined it properly, it should be expelled through the Idâ (left nostril). This destroys Vâta, pitta (bile) and phlegm and increases the digestive power (the gastric fire).

66.) kuṇḍalī bodhakaṃ kṣhipraṃ pavanaṃ sukhadaṃ hitam | brahma-nāḍī-mukhe saṃstha-kaphādy-arghala-nāśanam

It quickly awakens the Kundalinî, purifies the system, gives pleasure, and is beneficial. It destroys phlegm and the impurities accumulated at the entrance of the Brahma Nâdî.

**67.) samyaghghātra-samudbhūta-ghrant-
hi-traya-vibhedakam ǀ viśeṣheṇaiva kartavy-
aṃ bhastrākhyaṃ kumbhakaṃ tvidam**

*This Bhastrikâ should be performed plentifully, for it
breaks the three knots: Brahma granthi (in the chest),
Visnu granthi (in the throat), and Rudra granthi
(between the eyebrows) of the body.*

**68.) atha bhrāmarī
veghādghoṣhaṃ pūrakaṃ bhṛnggha-nādaṃ
bhṛngghī-nādaṃ rechakaṃ manda-mandam ǀ
yoghīndrāṇamevamabhyāsa-yoghāch chitte
jātā kāchidānanda-līlā**

The Bhrâmari.

*By filling the air with force, making noise like Bhringi
(wasp), and expelling it slowly, making noise in the same
way; this practice causes a sort of ecstacy in the minds of
Yogîndras.*

**69.) atha mūrchchā
pūrakānte ghāḍhataraṃ baddhvā jālandharaṃ
śanaiḥ ǀ rechayenmūrchchākhyeyaṃ ma-
no-mūrchchā sukha-pradā**

The Mûrchhâ.

Closing the passages with Jâlandhar Bandha firmly at the end of Pûraka, and expelling the air slowly, is called Mûrchhâ, from its causing the mind to swoon and giving comfort.

70.) atha plāvinī
antaḥ pravartitodāra-mārutāpūritodaraḥ |
payasyaghādhe|api sukhātplavate padma-pa-
travat

The Plâvinî.

When the belly is filled with air and the inside of the body is filled to its utmost with air, the body floats on the deepest water, like the leaf of a lotus.

71.) prāṇāyāmastridhā prokto recha-pūra-
ka-kumbhakaiḥ | sahitaḥ kevalaścheti kum-
bhako dvividho mataḥ

Considering Pûraka (Filling), Rechaka (expelling) and Kumbhaka (confining), Prânâyâma is of three kinds, but considering it accompanied by Pûraka and Rechaka, and without these, it is of two kinds only, i.e., Sahita (with) and Kevala (alone).

72.) yāvatkevala-siddhiḥ syātsahitaṃ tāvada-
bhyaset | rechakaṃ pūrakaṃ muktvā suk-
haṃ yadvāyu-dhāraṇam

*Exercise in Sahita should be continued till success in
Kevala is gained. This latter is simply confining the air
with ease, without Rechaka and Pûraka.*

73.) prāṇāyāmo|ayamityuktaḥ sa vai keva-
la-kumbhakaḥ | kumbhake kevale siddhe
recha-pūraka-varjite

*In the practice of Kevala Prânâyâma when it can be
performed successfully without Rechaka and Pûraka,
then it is called Kevala Kumbhaka.*

74.) na tasya durlabhaṃ kiṃchittriṣhu lo-
keṣhu vidyate | śaktaḥ kevala-kumbhena
yatheṣhṭaṃ vāyu-dhāraṇāt

*There is nothing in the three worlds which may be
difficult to obtain for him who is able to keep the air
confined according to pleasure, by means of Kevala
Kumbhaka.*

75.) rāja-yogha-padaṃ chāpi labhate nātra
saṃśayaḥ | kumbhakātkuṇḍalī-bodhaḥ

**kuṇḍalī-bodhato bhavet ǀ anarghalā suṣ-
humṇā cha haṭha-siddhiścha jāyate**

*He obtains the position of Râja Yoga undoubtedly. Kun-
dalinî awakens by Kumbhaka, and by its awakening,
Susumnâ becomes free from impurities.*

**76.) haṭhaṃ vinā rājayogho rāja-yoghaṃ vinā
haṭhaḥ ǀ na sidhyati tato yughmamāniṣhpat-
teḥ samabhyaset**

*No success in Râja Yoga without Hatha Yoga, and no
success in Hatha Yoga without Râja Yoga. One should,
therefore, practise both of these well, till complete success
is gained.*

**77.) kumbhaka-prāṇa-rodhānte kuryāchchit-
taṃ nirāśrayam ǀ evamabhyāsa-yoghena
rāja-yogha-padaṃ vrajet**

*On the completion of Kumbhaka, the mind should be
given rest. By practising in this way one is raised to the
position of (succeeds in getting) Râja Yoga.*

**78.) vapuḥ kṛśatvaṃ vadane prasannatā nā-
da-sphuṭatvaṃ nayane sunirmale ǀ aroghatā
bindu-jayoǀaghni-dīpanaṃ nāḍī-viśuddhir-
haṭha-siddhi-lakṣhaṇam**

Indications of success in the practice of Hatha Yoga.

When the body becomes lean, the face glows with delight, Anâhatanâda manifests, and eyes are clear, body is healthy, bindu under control, and appetite increases, then one should know that the Nâdîs are purified and success in Hatha Yoga is approaching.

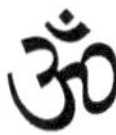

iti haṭha-pradīpikāyāṃ dvitīyopadeśaḥ

End of Chapter II.

Chapter 3

MUDRAS

Tṛtīyopadeśah

**1.) sa-śaila-vana-dhātrīṇāṃ yathād-
hāro|ahi-nāyakaḥ I sarveṣhāṃ yogha-tan-
trāṇāṃ tathādhāro hi kuṇḍalī**

*As the chief of the snakes is the support of the earth with
all the mountains and forests on it, so all the Tantras
(Yoga practices) rest on the Kundalinî. (The Vertebral
column.)*

**2.) suptā ghuru-prasādena yadā jāgharti
kuṇḍalī I tadā sarvāṇi padmāni bhidyante
ghranthayo|api cha**

*When the sleeping Kundalinî awakens by favour of a
guru, then all the lotuses (in the six chakras or centres)
and all the knots are pierced through.*

**3.) prāṇasya śūnya-padavī tadā rājapathāy-
ate I tadā chittaṃ nirālambaṃ tadā kālasya
vañchanam**

*Susumnâ (Sûnya Padavî) becomes a main road for the
passage of Prâna, and the mind then becomes free from*

all connections (with its objects of enjoyments) and Death is then evaded.

4.) suṣhumṇā śūnya-padavī brahma-randhraḥ mahāpathaḥ I śmaśānaṃ śāmbhavī mad-hya-mārghaśchetyeka-vāchakāḥ

Susumnâ, Sunya Padavî, Brahma Randhra, Mahâ Patha, Śmaśâna, Śambhavî, Madhya Mârga, are names of one and the same thing.

5.) tasmātsarva-prayatnena prabodhayi-tumīśvarīm I brahma-dvāra-mukhe suptāṃ mudrābhyāsaṃsamācharet

In order, therefore, to awaken this goddess, who is sleeping at the entrance of Brahma Dwâra (the great door), mudrâs should be practised well.

6.) mahāmudrā mahābandho mahāvedhaścha khecharī I uḍḍīyānaṃ mūlabandhaścha bandho jālandharābhidhaḥ

The mudrâs.

Mahâ Mudrâ, Mahâ Bandha, Mahâ Vedha, Khecharî, Uddiyâna Bandha, Mûla Bandha, Jâlandhara Bandha.

**7.) karaṇī viparītākhyā vajrolī śakti-chālanam
I idaṃ hi mudrā-daśakaṃ jarā-maraṇa-nāśa-
nam**

*Viparîta Karanî, Vajroli, and Śakti Châlana. These are
the ten Mudrâs which annihilate old age and death.*

**8.) ādināthoditaṃ divyamaṣhṭaiśva-
rya-pradāyakam I vallabhaṃ sarva-sidd-
hānāṃ durlabhaṃ marutāmapi**

*They have been explained by Âdi Nâtha (Śiva) and give
eight kinds of divine wealth. They are loved by all the
Siddhas and are hard to attain even by the Marutas.*

*Note.—The eight Aiśwaryas are: Animâ (becoming
small, like an atom), Mahimâ (becoming great, like
âkâs, by drawing in atoms of Prakriti), Garimâ (light
things, like cotton becoming very heavy like mountains.)*

*Prâpti (coming within easy reach of everything; as
touching the moon with the little finger, while standing
on the earth.)*

*Prâkâmya (non-resistance to the desires, as entering the
earth like water.)*

Îsatâ (mastery over matter and objects made of it.)

Vaśitwa (controlling the animate and inanimate objects.)

9.) ghopanīyaṃ prayatnena yathā ratna-ka-raṇḍakam I kasyachinnaiva vaktavyaṃ kula-strī-surataṃ yathā

These Mudrâs should be kept secret by every means, as one keeps one's box of jewellery, and should, on no account be told to any one, just as husband and wife keep their dealings secret.

10.) atha mahā-mudrā
pāda-mūlena vāmena yoniṃ sampīḍya dakṣhiṇām I prasāritam padaṃ kṛtvā karābhyāṃ dhārayeddṛḍham

The mahâ mudrâ.

Pressing the Yoni (perineum) with the heel of the left foot, and stretching forth the right foot, its toe should be grasped by the thumb and first finger.

11+12.) kaṇṭhe bandhaṃ samāropya dhāray-edvāyumūrdhvataḥ I yathā daṇḍa-hataḥ

**sarpo daṇḍākāraḥ prajāyate
ṛjvībhūtā tathā śaktiḥ kuṇḍalī sahasā bhavet
I tadā sā maraṇāvasthā jāyate dviputāśrayā**

*By stopping the throat (by Jâlandhara Bandha) the air
is drawn in from the outside and carried down. Just as a
snake struck with a stick becomes straight like a stick, in
the same way, śakti (susumnâ) becomes straight at once.
Then the Kundalinî, becoming as it were dead, and,*

*leaving both the Idâ and the Pingalâ, enters the su-
sumnâ (the middle passage). 11-12.*

**13.) tataḥ śanaiḥ śanaireva rechayennaiva ve-
ghataḥ I mahā-mudrāṃ cha tenaiva vadanti
vibudhottamāḥ**

*It should be expelled then, slowly only and not violently.
For this very reason, the best of the wise men call it the
Mahâ Mudrâ. This Mahâ Mudrâ has been propounded
by great masters.*

**14.) iyaṃ khalu mahāmudrā mahā-siddhaiḥ
pradarśitā I mahā-kleśādayo doṣhāḥ kṣhīy-
ante maraṇādayaḥ I mahā-mudrāṃ cha
tenaiva vadanti vibudhottamāḥ**

Great evils and pains, like death, are destroyed by it, and for this reason wise men call it the Mahâ Mudrâ.

15.) chandrāngghe tu samabhyasya sūryāngghe punarabhyaset I yāvat-tulyā bhavetsangkhyā tato mudrāṃ visarjayet

Having practised with the left nostril, it should be practised with the right one; and, when the number on both sides becomes equal, then the mudrâ should be discontinued.

16.) na hi pathyamapathyaṃ vā rasāḥ sar-ve|api nīrasāḥ I api bhuktaṃ viṣhaṃ ghoraṃ pīyūṣhamapi jīryati

There is nothing wholesome or injurious; for the practice of this mudrâ destroys the injurious effects of all the rasas (chemicals). Even the deadliest of poisons, if taken, acts like nectar.

17.) kṣhaya-kuṣhṭha-ghudāvarta-ghulmājīrṇa-puroghamāḥ I tasya doṣhāḥ kṣhayam yānti mahāmudrāṃ tu yo|abhyaset

Consumption, leprosy, prolapsus anii, colic, and the diseases due to indigestion, all these irregularities are removed by the practice of this Mahâ Mudrâ.

18.) kathiteyaṃ mahāmudrā mahā-siddhi-karā nṛṇām | ghopanīyā prayatnena na deyā yasya kasyachit

This Mahâ Mudrâ has been described as the giver of great success (Siddhi) to men. It should be kept secret by every effort, and not revealed to any and everyone.

19.) atha mahā-bandhaḥ
pārṣhṇiṃ vāmasya pādasya yoni-sthāne niyo-jayet | vāmorūpari saṃsthāpya dakṣhiṇaṃ charaṇaṃ tathā

The Mahâ Bandha.

Press the left heel to the perineum and place the right foot on the left thigh.

20.) pūrayitvā tato vāyuṃ hṛdaye chubukaṃ dṛḍham | niṣhpīḍyaṃ vāyumākuñchya ma-no-madhye niyojayet

Fill in the air, keeping the chin firm against the chest, and, having pressed the air, the mind should he fixed on the middle of the eyebrows or in the susumnâ (the spine).

**21.) dhārayitvā yathā-śakti rechayedani-
laṃ śanaiḥ I savyāngghe tu samabhyasya
dakṣhāngghe punarabhyaset**

*Having kept it confined so long as possible, it should
be expelled slowly. Having practised on the left side, it
should be practised on the right side.*

**22.) matamatra tu keṣhāṃchitkaṇṭha-band-
haṃ vivarjayet I rāja-danta-stha-jihvāyā
bandhaḥ śasto bhavediti**

*Some are of opinion that the closing of throat is not ne-
cessary here, for keeping the tongue pressed against the
roots of the upper teeth makes a good bandha (stop).*

**23.) ayaṃ tu sarva-nāḍīnāmūrdhvaṃ gha-
ti-nirodhakaḥ I ayaṃ khalu mahā-bandho
mahā-siddhi-pradāyakaḥ**

*This stops the upward motion of all the Nâdîs. Verily
this Mahâ Bandha is the giver of great Siddhis.*

**24.) kāla-pāśa-mahā-bandha-vimochana-
vichakṣhaṇaḥ I triveṇī-sangghamaṃ dhatte
kedāraṃ prāpayenmanaḥ**

This Mahâ Bandha is the most skilful means for cutting away the snares of death. It brings about the conjunction of the Trivenî (Idâ, Pingalâ and Susumnâ) and carries the mind to Kedâr (the space between the eyebrows, which is the seat of Śiva).

25.) rūpa-lāvaṇya-sampannā yathā strī puruṣaṃ vinā | maha-mudrā-mahā-band-hau niṣhphalau vedha-varjitau

As beauty and loveliness, do not avail a woman without husband, so the Mahâ Mudrâ and the Mahâ-Bandha are useless without the Mahâ Vedha.

26.) atha mahā-vedhaḥ mahā-bandha-sthito yoghī kṛtvā pūrakame-ka-dhīḥ | vāyūnāṃ ghatimāvṛtya nibhṛtaṃ kaṇṭha-mudrayā

The Mahâ Vedha.

Sitting with Mahâ Bandha, the Yogî should fill in the air and keep his mind collected. The movements of the Vâyus (Prâna and Apâna) should be stopped by closing the throat.)

**27.) sama-hasta-yugho bhūmau sphichau
sanāḍayechchanaiḥ | puṭa-dvayamatikramya
vāyuḥ sphurati madhyaghaḥ**

*Resting both the hands equally on the ground, he should
raise himself a little and strike his buttocks against the
ground gently. The air, leaving both the passages (Idâ
and Pingalâ), starts into the middle one.*

**28.) soma-sūryāghni-sambandho jāyate
chāmṛtāya vai | mṛtāvasthā samutpannā tato
vāyuṃ virechayet**

*The union of the Idâ and the Pingalâ is effected, in order
to bring about immortality. When the air becomes as it
were dead (by leaving its course through the Idâ and the
Pingalâ) (i.e., when it has been kept confined), then it
should be expelled.*

**29.) mahā-vedho|ayamabhyāsānmahā-sidd-
hi-pradāyakaḥ | valī-palita-vepa-ghnaḥ sevya-
te sādhakottamaiḥ**

*The practice of this Mahâ Vedha, the giver of great Sidd-
his, destroys old age, grey hair, and shaking of the body,
and therefore it is practised by the best masters.*

30.) etattrayaṃ mahā-ghuhyaṃ jarā-mṛtyu-vināśanam I vahni-vṛddhi-karaṃ chaiva hyaṇimādi-ghuṇa-pradam

These THREE are the great secrets. They are the destroyers of old age and death, increase the appetite, confer the accomplishments of Anima, etc.

31.) aṣhṭadhā kriyate chaiva yāme yāme dine dine I puṇya-saṃbhāra-sandhāya pāpaugha-bhiduraṃ sadā I samyak-śikṣhāvatāmevaṃ svalpaṃ prathama-sādhanam

They should, be practised in 8 ways, daily and hourly. They increase collection of good actions and lessen the evil ones. People, instructed well, should begin their practice, little by little, first.

32.) atha khecharī
kapāla-kuhare jihvā praviṣhṭā viparītaghā I bhruvorantarghatā dṛṣhṭirmudrā bhavati khecharī

The Khechari.

The Khechari Mudrâ is accomplished by thrusting the tongue into the gullet, by turning it over itself, and keeping the eyesight in the middle of the eyebrows.

**33.) chedana-chālana-dohaiḥ kalāṃ kra-
meṇātha vardhayettāvat I sā yāvad-
bhrū-madhyaṃ spṛśati tadā khecharī-siddhiḥ**

*To accomplish this, the tongue is lengthened by cutting
the frænum linguæ, moving, and pulling it. When it can
touch the space between the eyebrows, then Khechari
can be accomplished.*

**34.) snuhī-patra-nibhaṃ śastraṃ sutīkṣhṇaṃ
snighdha-nirmalam I samādāya tatastena
roma-mātraṃ samuchchinet**

*Taking a sharp, smooth, and clean instrument, of the
shape of a cactus leaf, the frænum of the tongue should
be cut a little (as much as a hair's thickness), at a time.*

**35.) tataḥ saindhava-pathyābhyāṃ
chūrṇitābhyāṃ pragharṣhayet I punaḥ sap-
ta-dine prāpte roma-mātraṃ samuchchinet**

*Then rock salt and yellow myrobalan (both powdered)
should be rubbed in. On the 7th day, it should again be
cut a hair's breadth.*

**36.) evaṃ krameṇa ṣhaṇ-māsaṃ nityaṃ yuk-
taḥ samācharet I ṣhaṇmāsādrasanā-mūla-
śirā-bandhaḥ praṇaśyati**

One should go on doing thus, regularly for six months. At the end of six months, the frænum of the tongue will be completely cut.

37.) kalāṃ parāngmukhīṃ kṛtvā tripathe pariyojayet I sā bhavetkhecharī mudrā vyo-ma-chakraṃ taduchyate

Turning the tongue upwards, it is fixed on the three ways (œsophagus, windpipe and palate.) Thus it makes the Khechari Mudrâ, and is called the Vyoma Chakra.

38.) rasanāmūrdhvaghāṃ kṛtvā kṣhaṇārd-hamapi tiṣhṭhati I viṣhairvimuchyate yoghī vyādhi-mṛtyu-jarādibhiḥ

The Yogî who sits for a minute turning his tongue upwards, is saved from poisons, diseases, death, old age, etc.

39.) na rogho maraṇaṃ tandrā na nidrā na kṣ-hudhā tṛṣhā I na cha mūrchchā bhavettasya yo mudrāṃ vetti khecharīm

He who knows the Khechari Mudrâ is not afflicted with disease, death, sloth, sleep, hunger, thirst, and swooning.

40.) pīḍyate na sa roghena lipyate na cha

karmaṇā | bādhyate na sa kālena yo mudrāṃ
vetti khecharīm

*He who knows the Khechari Mudrâ, is not troubled by
diseases, is not stained with karmas, and is not snared
by time.*

41.) chittaṃ charati khe yasmājjihvā charati khe ghatā | tenaiṣā khecharī nāma mudrā siddhairnirūpitā

*The Siddhas have devised this Khechari Mudrâ from
the fact that the mind and the tongue reach âkâśa by its
practice.*

42.) khecharyā mudritaṃ yena vivaraṃ lam-bikordhvataḥ | na tasya kṣharate binduḥ kāminyāḥ śleṣhitasya cha

*If the hole behind the palate be stopped with Khechari
by turning the tongue upwards, then bindu cannot leave
its place even if a woman were embraced.*

43.) chalito|api yadā binduḥ samprāpto yo-ni-maṇḍalam | vrajatyūrdhvaṃ hṛtaḥ śaktyā nibaddho yoni-mudrayā

Even when there is movement of the bindu and it enters

*the genitals, it is seized by closing the perineum and is
taken upward.*

44.) ūrdhva-jihvaḥ sthiro bhūtvā somapānaṃ karoti yaḥ | māsārdhena na sandeho mṛtyuṃ jayati yoghavit

*If the Yogî drinks Somarasa (juice) by sitting with the
tongue turned backwards and mind concentrated, there
is no doubt he conquers death within 15 days.*

45.) nityaṃ soma-kalā-pūrṇaṃ śarīraṃ yasya yoghinaḥ | takṣhakeṇāpi daṣhṭasya viṣhaṃ tasya na sarpati

*The yogi's body is forever full of the moon's nectar. Even
if he is bitten by the king of snakes (Takshaka), he is not
poisoned*

46.) indhanāni yathā vahnistaila-varti cha dī-pakaḥ | tathā soma-kalā-pūrṇaṃ dehī dehaṃ na muñchati

*Just as fuel kindles fire and oil a lamp, so the indweller
of the body does not vacate while the body is full of the
moon's nectar*

47.) ghomāṃsaṃ bhakṣhayennityaṃ pibe-damara-vāruṇīm | kulīnaṃ tamahaṃ manye chetare kula-ghātakāḥ

By constant swallowing of the tongue he can drink amaravaruni. I consider him of high lineage (heritage). Others destroy the heritage.

48.) gho-śabdenoditā jihvā tatpraveśo hi tāluni | gho-māṃsa-bhakṣhaṇaṃ tattu mahā-pātaka-nāśanam

The word 'go' means tongue (and also means cow). When it enters into the upper palate, it is 'eating the flesh of the cow.' It (khechari) destroys the great sins.

49.) jihvā-praveśa-sambhūta-vahninotpāditaḥ khalu | chandrātsravati yaḥ sāraḥ sā syāda-mara-vāruṇī

When the tongue enters the cavity, indeed heat is produced and the man's nectar flows.

50.) chumbantī yadi lambikāghramaniśaṃ jihvā-rasa-syandinī sa-kṣhārā kaṭukām-la-dughdha-sadṛśī madhvājya-tulyā tathā | vyādhīnāṃ haraṇaṃ jarānta-karaṇaṃ

**śastrāghamodīraṇaṃ tasya syādamaratva-
maṣhṭa-ghuṇitaṃ siddhāngghanākarṣhaṇam**

*When the tongue constantly presses the cavity, the
moon's nectar (flows and) has a saline, pungent and
acidic flavor. It is like (the consistency of) milk, ghee,
honey. Fatal diseases, old age and weapons are warded
off. From that, immortality and the eight siddhis or
perfections manifest.*

**51.) ūrdvhāsyo rasanāṃ niyamya vivare śak-
tiṃ parāṃ chintayan I utkallola-kalā-jalaṃ
cha vimalaṃ dhārāmayaṃ yaḥ piben nirvyād-
hiḥ sa mṛṇāla-komala-vapuryoghī chiraṃ
jīvati**

*Fluid drips into the sixteen petalled lotus (vishuddhi
chakra) when the tongue is inserted into the upper
throat cavity; the paramshakti (kundalini) is released
and one becomes concentrated in that (experience which
ensues). The yogi who drinks the pure stream of nectar
is freed from disease, has longevity, and has a body as
soft and as beautiful as a lotus stem.*

**52.) yatprāleyaṃ prahita-suṣhiraṃ
meru-mūrdhāntara-sthaṃ tasmiṃstattvaṃ
pravadati sudhīstan-mukhaṃ nimnaghānām**

I chandrātsārah sravati vapushastena mṛty-
urnarāṇāṃ tadbadhnīyātsukaraṇamadho
nānyathā kāya-siddhiḥ

*The nectar is secreted from the topmost part of the
Meru (Sushumna), the fountainhead of the nadis. He
who has pure intellect can know the Truth therein. The
nectar, which is the essence of the body, flows out from
the moon and hence death ensues. Therefore khechari
mudra should be practiced, otherwise perfection of the
body cannot be attained.*

53.) suṣhiraṃ jñāna-janakaṃ pañcha-sro-
taḥ-samanvitam I tiṣhṭhate khecharī mudrā
tasminśūnye nirañjane

*Five nadis convene in this cavity and it is the source of
knowledge. Khechari should be established in that void,
untainted (by ignorance).*

54.) ekaṃ sṛṣhṭimayaṃ bījamekā mudrā cha
khecharī I eko devo nirālamba ekāvasthā
manonmanī

*There is only one seed of creation and one mudra –
khechari; one deva independent of everything and one
state – manonmani.*

55.) atha uḍḍīyāna-bandhaḥ

baddho yena sushumṇāyāṃ prāṇastūḍḍīyate
yataḥ | tasmāduḍḍīyanākhyo|ayaṃ yog-
hibhiḥ samudāhṛtaḥ

The Uddiyâna bandha.

Uddiyana bandha is so-called by the yogis because
through its practice the prana (is concentrated at one
point and) rises through sushumna.

56.) uḍḍīnaṃ kurute yasmādaviśrāntaṃ
mahā-khaghaḥ | uḍḍīyānaṃ tadeva syāttava
bandho|abhidhīyate

The bandha described is called the rising or flying band-
ha, because through its practice, the great bird (shakti)
flies upward with ease.

57.) udare paśchimaṃ tānaṃ nābherūrdh-
vaṃ cha kārayet | uḍḍīyāno hyasau bandho
mṛtyu-mātanggha-kesarī

Pulling the abdomen back in and making the navel rise
is uddiyana bandha. It is the lion which conquers the
elephant, death.

58.) uḍḍīyānaṃ tu sahajaṃ ghuruṇā kathitaṃ sadā I abhyasetsatataṃ yastu vṛddho|api taruṇāyate

Uddiyana is easy when practiced as told by the guru. Even an old person can become young when it is done regularly.

59.) nābherūrdhvamadhaśchāpi tānaṃ kuryātprayatnataḥ I ṣhaṇmāsamabhyasen-mṛtyuṃ jayatyeva na saṃśayaḥ

The region above and below the navel should be drawn backward with effort. There is no doubt that after six months of practice, death is conquered.

60.) sarveṣhāmeva bandhānāṃ uttamo hyuḍḍīyānakaḥ I uḍḍiyāne dṛḍhe bandhe muktiḥ svābhāvikī bhavet

Of all the bandhas, uddiyana is the best. Once it is mastered, mukti or liberation occurs spontaneously.

61.) atha mūla-bandhaḥ pārṣhṇi-bhāghena sampīḍya yonimākuñchay-edghudam I apānamūrdhvamākṛṣhya mūla-bandho|abhidhīyate

The Moola bhanda.

Pressing the perineum/vagina with the heel and contracting the rectum so that the apana vayu moves upward is moola bandha.

62.) adho-ghatimapānaṃ vā ūrdhvaghaṃ kurute balāt l ākuñchanena taṃ prāhurmūla-bandhaṃ hi yoghinaḥ

By contracting the perineum the downward moving apana vayu is forced to go upward. Yogis call this moola bandha.

63.) ghudaṃ pārṣhṇyā tu sampīḍya vāyumākuñchayedbalāt l vāraṃ vāraṃ yathā chordhvaṃ samāyāti samīraṇaḥ

Press the heel firmly against the rectum and contract forcefully and repeatedly, so that the vital energy rises.

64.) prāṇāpānau nāda-bindū mūla-bandhena chaikatām l ghatvā yoghasya saṃsiddhiṃ yachchato nātra saṃśayaḥ

There is no doubt that by practicing moola bandha, prana/apana and nada/bindu are united, and total perfection attained.

65.) apāna-prāṇayoraikyaṃ kṣhayo mūtra-purīṣhayoḥ | yuvā bhavati vṛddho|api satataṃ mūla-bandhanāt

With constant practice of moola bandha, prana and apana unite, urine and stool are decreased and even an old person becomes young.

66.) apāna ūrdhvaghe jāte prayāte vahni-maṇḍalam | tadānala-śikhā dīrghā jāyate vāyunāhatā

Apana moves up into the region of fire (manipura chakra, the navel center), then the flames of the fire grow, being fanned by apana vayu.

67.) tato yāto vahny-apānau prāṇamuṣhṇa-svarūpakam | tenātyanta-pradīptastu jvalano dehajastathā

Then, when apana and the fin meet with prana, which is itself hot, the heat in the body is intensified.

68.) tena kuṇḍalinī suptā santaptā samprabudhyate | daṇḍāhatā bhujangghīva niśvasya ṛjutāṃ vrajet

Through this, the sleeping kundalini is aroused by the extreme heat and it straightens itself just as a serpent beaten with a stick straightens and hisses.

69.) bilaṃ praviṣhṭeva tato brahma-nāḍyaṃ taraṃ vrajet I tasmānnityaṃ mūla-bandhaḥ kartavyo yoghibhiḥ sadā

Just as a snake enters its hole, so kundalini goes into brahma nadi. Therefore the yogi must always perform moola bandha.

70.) atha jalandhara-bandhaḥ kaṇṭhamākuñchya hṛdaye sthāpayechchibu- kaṃ dṛḍham I bandho jālandharākhyoḷayaṃ jarā-mṛtyu-vināśakaḥ

The Jâlandhara Bandha.

Contracting the throat by bringing the chin to the chest is the bandha called jalandhara. It destroys old age and death.

71.) badhnāti hi sirājālamadho-ghāmi nabho-jalam I tato jālandharo bandhaḥ kaṇṭha-duḥkhaugha-nāśanaḥ

That is jalandhara bandha which catches the flow of nectar in the throat. It destroys all throat ailments.

72.) jālandhare kṛte bandhe kaṇṭha-saṃko-cha-lakṣhaṇe | na pīyūṣhaṃ patatyaghnau na cha vāyuḥ prakupyati

Having done jalandhara bandha by contracting the throat, the nectar does not fall into the gastric fire and the prana is not agitated.

73.) kaṇṭha-saṃkochanenaiva dve nāḍyau stambhayeddṝḍham | madhya-chakramidaṃ jñeyaṃ ṣhoḍaśādhāra-bandhanam

The two Nâdîs should be stopped firmly by contracting the throat. This is called the middle circuit or centre (Madhya Chakra), and it stops the 16 âdhâras (i.e., vital parts).

Note.

The sixteen vital parts mentioned by renowned Yogîs are the (1) thumbs, (2) ankles, (3) knees, (4) thighs, (5) the prepuce, (6) organs of generation, (17) the navel, (8) the heart, (9) the neck, (10) the throat, (11) the palate, (12) the nose, (13) the middle of the eyebrows, (14) the forehead, (15) the head and (16) the Brahma randhra.

74.) mūla-sthānaṃ samākuñchya uḍḍiyānaṃ tu kārayet | iḍāṃ cha pingghalāṃ baddhvā vāhayetpaśchime pathi

By drawing up the mûlasthâna (anus,) Uddiyâna Bandha should be performed. The flow of the air should be directed to the Susumnâ, by closing the Idâ, and the Pingalâ. 73.

75.) anenaiva vidhānena prayāti pavano layam | tato na jāyate mṛtyurjarā-roghādikaṃ tathā

The Prâna becomes calm and latent by this means, and thus there is no death, old age, disease, etc.

76.) bandha-trayamidaṃ śreṣhṭhaṃ mahā-siddhaiścha sevitam | sarveṣhāṃ haṭha-tantrāṇāṃ sādhanaṃ yoghino viduḥ

These three Bandhas are the best of all and have been practised by the masters. Of all the means of success in the Hatha Yoga, they are known to the Yogîs as the chief ones.

77.) yatkiṃchitsravate chandrādamṛtaṃ divya-rūpiṇaḥ | tatsarvaṃ ghrasate sūryastena piṇḍo jarāyutaḥ

*That nectar which flows from the moon has the quality
of endowing enlightenment, but it is completely consumed by the sun, incurring old age.*

78.) atha viparīta-karaṇī mudrā
tatrāsti karaṇaṃ divyaṃ sūryasya muk-
ha-vañchanam I ghurūpadeśato jñeyaṃ na tu
śāstrārtha-koṭibhiḥ

The Viparîta Karani.

*There is a wonderful means by which the nectar is
averted from falling into the opening of the sun. This is
obtained by the guru's instructions and not from the
hundreds of shastras (treatises).*

79.) ūrdhva-nābheradhastālorūrdhvaṃ
bhānuradhaḥ śaśī I karaṇī viparītākhā ghu-
ru-vākyena labhyate

*With the navel region above and the palate below, the
sun is above and the moon below. It is called vipareeta
karani, the reversing process. When given by the guru's
instructions it is fruitful.*

80.) nityamabhyāsa-yuktasya jaṭharāghni-vi-
vardhanī I āhāro bahulastasya sampādyaḥ
sādhakasya cha

Digestion is strengthened by continual, regular practice and therefore, the practitioner should always have sufficient food.

81.) alpāhāro yadi bhavedaghnirdahati tat-kṣhaṇāt I adhaḥ-śirāśchordhva-pādaḥ kṣhaṇaṃ syātprathame dine

If one takes only a little food, the heat produced by the digestion will destroy the system. Therefore, on the first day, one should only stay a moment with the feet up and head down.

82.) kṣhaṇāchcha kiṃchidadhikamabhya-sechcha dine dine I valitaṃ palitaṃ chaiva ṣhaṇmāsordhvaṃ na dṝśyate I yāma-mātraṃ tu yo nityamabhyasetsa tu kālajit

The practice should be done daily, gradually increasing the duration. After six months of practice, grey hairs and wrinkles become inconspicuous. One who practices it for yama (three hours conquers death.

83.) atha vajrolī svechchayā vartamāno|api yoghoktairniy-amairvinā I vajrolīṃ yo vijānāti sa yoghī siddhi-bhājanam

The Vajrolî.

Even anyone living a free lifestyle without the formal rules of yoga, if he practices vajroli well, that yogi becomes a recipient of siddhis (perfections).

84.) tatra vastu-dvayaṃ vakṣhye durlabhaṃ yasya kasyachit ǀ kṣhīraṃ chaikaṃ dvitīyaṃ tu nārī cha vaśa-vartinī

There are two things hard to obtain, one is milk and the second is a woman who can act according to your will.

85.) mehanena śanaiḥ samyaghūrdh-vākuñchanamabhyaset ǀ puruṣhoǀapyathavā nārī vajrolī-siddhimāpnuyāt

By practicing gradual upward contractions during the emission in intercourse, any man or woman achieves perfection of vajroli.

86.) yatnataḥ śasta-nālena phūtkāraṃ vaj-ra-kandare ǀ śanaiḥ śanaiḥ prakurvīta vāyu-saṃchāra-kāraṇāt

By slowly drawing in air through a prescribed tube inserted into the urethra of the penis, gradually air and prana traverse into the vajra kanda.

**87.) nārī-bhaghe padad-bindumabhyāsenord-
hvamāharet I chalitaṃ cha nijaṃ bindumūrd-
hvamākṛṣhya rakṣhayet**

*The bindu (semen) that is about to fall into the woman's
vagina should be made to move upwards with practice.
And if it falls, the semen and the woman's fluid should
be conserved by drawing it up.*

**88.) evaṃ saṃrakṣhayedbinduṃ jayati
yoghavit I maraṇaṃ bindu-pātena jīvanaṃ
bindu-dhāraṇāt**

*Therefore, the knower of yoga conquers death by pre-
serving the bindu (semen). Release of the bindu means
death; conservation of semen is life.*

**89.) sughandho yoghino dehe jāyate bin-
du-dhāraṇāt I yāvadbinduḥ sthiro dehe
tāvatkāla-bhayaṃ kutaḥ**

*As long as the bindu/semen is steady in the body, then
where is the fear of death? The yogi's body smells pleasant by conserving the bindu/semen.*

**90.) chittāyattaṃ nṝṇāṃ śukraṃ śukrāyattaṃ
cha jīvitam I tasmāchchhukraṃ manaśchaiva
rakṣhaṇīyaṃ prayatnataḥ**

A man's semen can be controlled by the mind and control of semen is life giving. Therefore, his semen and mind should be controlled and conserved.

91.) r̥tumatyā rajo|apyevaṃ nijaṃ binduṃ ch rakṣhayet I meḍhreṇākarṣhayedūrdhvaṃ samyaghabhyāsa-yogha-vit

The knower of yoga, perfect in the practice, conserves his bindu and the woman's rajas by drawing it up through the generative organ.

92.) atha sahajoliḥ sahajoliśchāmarolirvajrolyā bheda ekataḥ I jale subhasma nikṣhipya daghdha-gho- maya-sambhavam

The Sahajolî.

Sahajoli and amaroli are separate techniques of vajroli. The ashes of burnt cow manure should be mixed with water.

93.) vajrolī-maithunādūrdhvaṃ strī-puṃsoḥ svānggha-lepanam I āsīnayoḥ sukhenaiva mukta-vyāpārayoḥ kṣhaṇāt

After performing vajroli during intercourse, (being in a

comfortable position), the man and woman should wipe
the ashes on specific parts of their bodies during the
leisure time.

94.) sahajoliriyaṃ proktā śraddheyā yog-hibhiḥ sadā | ayaṃ śubhakaro yogho bhog-ha-yukto|api muktidaḥ

It is called sahajoli and the yogis have complete faith
in it. This is very beneficial and enables enlightenment
through the combination of yoga and bhoga (sensual
involvement).

95.) ayaṃ yoghaḥ puṇyavatāṃ dhīrāṇāṃ tatt-va-darśinām | nirmatsarāṇāṃ vai sidhyenna tu matsara-śālinām

Verily this yoga is perfected by virtuous and well-con-
ducted men who have seen the truth and not those who
are selfish.

96.) atha amarolī pittolbaṇatvātprathamāmbu-dhārāṃ vihāya niḥsāratayāntyadhārām | niṣhevyate śīta-la-madhya-dhārā kāpālike khaṇḍamate|a-marolī

The Amarolî.

According to the Kapalika sect, amaroli is practiced by drinking the cool midstream of urine. The first part of the urine is left as it contains bile, and the last part is left as it does not contain goodness.

97.) amarīṃ yaḥ pibennityaṃ nasyaṃ kur-vandine dine | vajrolīmabhyasetsamyaksā-marolīti kathyate

One who drinks amari, takes it through the nose and practices vajroli, is said to be practicing amaroli.

98.) abhyāsānniḥsṛtāṃ chāndrīṃ vibhūtyā saha miśrayet | dhārayeduttamānggheṣhu divya-dṛṣhṭiḥ prajāyate

The practitioner should mix the semen with the ashes of burnt cow manure and wipe it on the upper parts of the body, it bestows divya drishti (clairvoyance or divine sight).

99.) puṃso binduṃ samākuñchya samyag-habhyāsa-pāṭavāt | yadi nārī rajo rakṣhed-vajrolyā sāpi yoghinī

If a woman practices vajroli and saves her rajas and the man's bindu by thorough contraction, she is a yogini.

100.) tasyāḥ kiṃchidrajo nāśaṃ na ghach-chati na saṃśayaḥ l tasyāḥ śarīre nādaścha bindutāmeva ghachchati

Without doubt, not even a little rajas is wasted through vajroli, the nada and bindu in the body become one.

101.) sa bindustadrajaśchaiva ekībhūya sva-dehaghau l vajroly-abhyāsa-yoghena sar-va-siddhiṃ prayachchataḥ

The bindu and that rajas in one's own body unite through the union by practice of vajroli, thus bestowing all perfections or siddhis.

102.) rakṣhedākuñchanādūrdhvaṃ yā rajaḥ sā hi yoghinī l atītānāghataṃ vetti khecharī cha bhaveddhruvam

She is verily a yogini who conserves her rajas by contracting and raising it. She knows past, present and future and becomes fixed in khechari (i.e. consciousness moves into the higher realm).

103.) deha-siddhiṃ cha labhate vaj-roly-abhyāsa-yoghataḥ | ayaṃ puṇya-karo yogho bhoghe bhukte | api muktidaḥ

By the yoga of vajroli practice, perfection of the body fructifies. This auspicious yoga even brings liberation alongside with sensual involvement (bhoga).

104.) atha śakti-chālanam kuṭilāngghī kuṇḍalinī bhujangghī śaktirīśvarī | kuṇḍalyarundhatī chaite śabdāḥ pa-ryāya-vāchakāḥ

The Śakti châlana.

Kutilangi, kundalini, bhujangi, shakti, ishwari, kundali, arundhati are all synonymous terms.

105.) udghāṭayetkapāṭaṃ tu yathā kuṃchi-kayā haṭhāt | kuṇḍalinyā tathā yoghī mokṣhadvāraṃ vibhedayet

Just as a door is opened with a key, similarly the yogi opens the door to liberation with kundalini.

106.) yena mārgheṇa ghantavyaṃ brahma-st-hānaṃ nirāmayam | mukhenāchchhādya tadvāraṃ prasuptā parameśvarī

The sleeping Parameshwari rests with her mouth closing that door, through which is the path to the knot of brahmasthana, the place beyond suffering.

107.) kandordhve kuṇḍalī śaktiḥ suptā mokṣhāya yoghinām | bandhanāya cha mūḍhānāṃ yastāṃ vetti sa yoghavit

The kundalini shakti sleeps above the kanda. This shakti is the means of liberation to the yogi and bondage for the ignorant.

One who knows this is the knower of yoga.

108.) kuṇḍalī kuṭilākārā sarpavatparikīrtitā | sā śaktiśchālitā yena sa mukto nātra saṃśay-aḥ

Kundalini is said to be coiled like a snake. **Without a doubt, one who makes that shakti flow obtains liberation.**

109.) ghanggghā-yamunayormadhye bāla-raṇḍāṃ tapasvinīm | balātkāreṇa ghṛhṇīyāt-tadviṣhṇoḥ paramaṃ padam

Between Ganga and Yamuna is the young widowed,

110.) iḍā bhaghavatī ghangghā pingghalā yamunā nadī । iḍā-pingghalayormadhye bālaraṇḍā cha kuṇḍalī

Ida is the holy Ganga, pingala the river Yamuna. Between ida and pingala in the middle is this young widow, kundalini.

111.) puchche praghṛhya bhujangghīṃ suptāmudbodhayechcha tām । nidrāṃ vihāya sā śaktirūrdhvamuttiṣhṭhate haṭhāt

By seizing the tail of kundalini serpent, she becomes very excited. Abandoning sleep that shakti is released and rises up.

112.) avasthitā chaiva phaṇāvatī sā prātaścha sāyaṃ praharārdha-mātram । prapūrya sūryātparidhāna-yuktyā praghṛhya nityaṃ parichālanīyā

Shakti Chalana Mudra.

Breathing in through the right nostril (pingala) the serpent (shakti) should be seized through kumbhaka

*and rotated constantly for an hour and a half, morning
and evening.*

113.) ūrdhvaṃ vitasti-mātram tu vistāram cha-
turangghulam I mṛdulam dhavalam proktam
veṣhṭitāmbara-lakṣhaṇam

*The kanda, situated above the anus, one hand span
high and four fingers breath wide, is soft and white as if
enveloped in cloth.*

114.) sati vajrāsane pādau karābhyāṃ dhāray-
eddṛḍham I ghulpha-deśa-samīpe cha kan-
dam tatra prapīḍayet

*Firmly seated in vajrasana, holding the ankles, one
should squeeze the kanda close to the anus.*

115.) vajrāsane sthito yoghī chālayitvā cha
kuṇḍalīm I kuryādanantaram bhastrām
kuṇḍalīmāśu bodhayet

*In the position of vajrasana, the yogi should move the
kundalini. Having done bhastrika pranayama the kundalini is soon aroused.*

116.) bhānorākuñchanam kuryātkuṇḍalīṃ

chālayettataḥ | mṛtyu-vaktra-ghatasyāpi tasya mṛtyu-bhayaṃ kutaḥ

Contracting the sun in manipura, kundalini should be moved. Even if such a person should be on the verge of death, where is the need to fear death?

117.) muhūrta-dvaya-paryantaṃ nirbhay-am chālanādasau | ūrdhvamākṛṣhyate kiṃchitsuṣhumṇāyāṃ samudghatā

By moving the kundalini fearlessly for an hour and a half, it is drawn into sushumna and rises up a little.

118.) tena kuṇdalinī tasyāḥ suṣhumṇāyā mukhaṃ dhruvam | jahāti tasmātprāṇo|ayaṃ suṣhumṇāṃ vrajati svataḥ

In this way, it is easy for kundalini to issue from the opening of sushumna. Thus the prana proceeds through sushumna of its own accord.

119.) tasmātsaṃchālayennityaṃ sukha-suptā-marundhatīm | tasyāḥ saṃchālanenaiva yoghī roghaiḥ pramuchyate

In that way the sleeping kundalini should be regularly

moved. By her regular movement, the yogi is freed from disease.

120.) yena saṃchālitā śaktiḥ sa yoghī siddhi-bhājanam | kimatra bahunoktena kālaṃ jayati līlayā

The yogi who moves the shakti regularly, enjoys perfection or siddhi. He easily conquers time and death. What more is there to say?

121.) brahmacharya-ratasyaiva nityaṃ hita-mitāśinaḥ | maṇḍalāddṛśyate siddhiḥ kuṇḍaly-abhyāsa-yoghinaḥ

One who enjoys being brahmacharya and always takes moderate diet and practices arousal of kundalini, achieves perfection in forty days.

122.) kuṇḍalīṃ chālayitvā tu bhastrāṃ kuryādviśeṣhataḥ | evamabhyasyato nityaṃ yamino yama-bhīḥ kutaḥ

Bhastrika pranayama with kumbhaka should specifically be practiced to activate kundalini. From where will the fear of death arise for a self- restrained practitioner who practices daily with regularity?

123.) dvā-saptati-sahasrāṇāṁ nāḍīnāṁ
mala-śodhane | kutaḥ prakṣhālanopāyaḥ
kuṇḍaly-abhyasanādṛte

*What other methods are there to cleanse the 72,000
nadis of dirt besides the practice of arousing kundalini?*

124.) iyaṁ tu madhyamā nāḍī dṛḍhābhyāsena
yoghinām | āsana-prāṇa-saṁyāma-mud-
rābhiḥ saralā bhavet

*This middle nadi, sushumna, easily becomes establis-
hed, (straight) by the yogi's persistent practice of asana,
pranayama, mudra and concentration.*

125.) abhyāse tu vinidrāṇāṁ mano dhṛtvā
samādhinā | rudrāṇī vā parā mudrā bhadrāṁ
siddhiṁ prayachchati

*For those who are alert and the mind one-pointed (dis-
ciplined) in samadhi, rudrani or shambhavi mudra is
the greatest mudra for bestowing perfection.*

126.) rāja-yoghaṁ vinā pṛthvī rāja-yoghaṁ
vinā niśā | rāja-yoghaṁ vinā mudrā vichitrā-
pi na śobhate

*The earth without raja yoga, night without raja yoga,
even the various mudras without raja yoga are useless,
i.e. not beautiful.*

127.) mārutasya vidhiṃ sarvaṃ mano-yuktaṃ samabhyaset I itaratra na kartavyā mano-vṛt-tirmanīṣhiṇā

*All the pranayama methods are to be done with a con-
centrated mind. The wise man should not let his mind
be involved in the modifications (vrittis).*

128.) iti mudrā daśa proktā ādināthena śam-bhunā I ekaikā tāsu yaminām mahā-sidd-hi-pradāyinī

*Thus the ten mudras have been told by Adinath,
Shambhu. Each one is the bestower of perfection to the
self-restrained.*

129.) upadeśaṃ hi mudrāṇāṃ yo datte sāmpradāyikam I sa eva śrī-ghuruḥ svāmī sākṣhādīśvara eva saḥ

*One who instructs mudra in the tradition of guru/disci-
ple is the true guru and form of Ishwara.*

130.) tasya vākya-paro bhūtvā mudrābhyā-

se samāhitaḥ | aṇimādi-ghuṇaiḥ sārdhaṃ labhate kāla-vañchanam

By following explicitly his (guru's) words, and practicing mudra; one obtains the qualities of anima, etc. and overcomes death/time

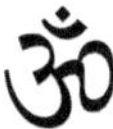

iti haṭha-pradīpikāyāṃ tṛtīyopadeśaḥ

End of chapter III, on the Exposition of the Mudrâs.

Chapter 4

Samadhi

Chaturthopadeśah

**1.) namaḥ śivāya ghurave nāda-bindu-kalāt-
mane | nirañjana-padaṃ yāti nityaṃ tatra
parāyaṇaḥ**

*Salutation to the Gurû, the dispenser of happiness to
all, appearing as Nâda, Vindû and Kalâ. One who is
devoted to Him, obtains the highest bliss.*

**2.) athedānīṃ pravakṣhyāmi samādhikra-
mamuttamam | mṛtyughnaṃ cha sukhopāy-
aṃ brahmānanda-karaṃ param**

*Now I will describe a regular method of attaining to
Samâdhi, which destroys death, is the means for obtaining happiness, and gives the Brahmânanda.*

**3+4.) rāja-yoghaḥ samādhiścha unmanī
cha manonmanī | amaratvaṃ layastattvaṃ
śūnyāśūnyaṃ paraṃ padam**

**amanaskaṃ tathādvaitaṃ nirālambaṃ nirañ-
janam | jīvanmuktiścha sahajā turyā chety-
eka-vāchakāḥ**

Raja Yogî, Samâdhi, Unmani, Mauonmanî, Amarativa, Laya, Tatwa, Sûnya, Aśûnya, Parama Pada, Amanaska, Adwaitama, Nirãlamba, Nirañjana, Jîwana Mukti, Sahajâ, Turyâ, are all synonymous.

5.) salile saindhavaṃ yadvatsāmyaṃ bhajati yoghataḥ | tathātma-manasoraikyaṃ samādhirabhidhīyate

As salt being dissolved in water becomes one with it, so when Âtmâ and mind become one, it is called Samâdhi.

6.) yadā saṃkṣhīyate prāṇo mānasaṃ cha pralīyate | tadā samarasatvaṃ cha samādhirabhidhīyate

When the Prâna becomes lean (vigourless) and the mind becomes absorbed, then their becoming equal is called Samâdhi.

7.) tat-samaṃ cha dvayoraikyaṃ jīvātma-paramātmanoḥ | pranaṣhṭa-sarva-sangkalpaḥ samādhiḥ so|abhidhīyate

This equality and oneness of the self and the ultra self, when all Sankalpas cease to exist, is called Samâdhi.

8.) rāja-yoghasya māhātmyaṃ ko vā jānāti tattvataḥ | jñānaṃ muktiḥ sthitiḥ siddhirghu-ru-vākyena labhyate

Or, who can know the true greatness of the Raja Yoga. Knowledge, mukti, condition, and Siddhîs can be learnt by instructions from a gurû alone.

9.) durlabho viṣhaya-tyāgho durlabhaṃ tattva-darśanam | durlabhā sahajāvasthā sad-ghuroḥ karuṇāṃ vinā

Indifference to worldly enjoyments is very difficult to obtain, and equally difficult is the knowledge of the Realities to obtain. It is very difficult to get the condition of Samâdhi, without the favour of a true guru.

10.) vividhairāsanaiḥ kubhairvichitraiḥ ka-raṇairapi | prabuddhāyāṃ mahā-śaktau prāṇaḥ śūnye pralīyate

By means of various postures and different Kumbha-kas, when the great power (Kundalî) awakens, then the Prâna becomes absorbed in Sûnya (Samâdhi).

11.) utpanna-śakti-bodhasya tyak-ta-niḥśeṣha-karmaṇaḥ | yoghinaḥ sa-hajāvasthā svayameva prajāyate

*The Yogî whose śakti has awakened, and who has reno-
unced all actions, attains to the condition of Samâdhi,
without any effort.*

12.) suṣhumṇā-vāhini prāṇe śūnye viśati mānase I tadā sarvāṇi karmāṇi nirmūlayati yoghavit

*When the Prâna flows in the Susumnâ, and the mind
has entered śûnya, then the Yogî is free from the effects
of Karmas.*

13.) amarāya namastubhyaṃ so|api kālast-vayā jitaḥ I patitaṃ vadane yasya jaghade-tachcharācharam

*O Immortal one (that is, the yogi who has attained to
the condition of Samâdhi), I salute thee! Even death
itself, into whose mouth the whole of this movable and
immovable world has fallen, has been conquered by
thee.*

14.) chitte samatvamāpanne vāyau vraja-ti madhyame I tadāmarolī vajrolī sahajolī prajāyate

Amarolî, Vajrolî and Sahajolî are accomplished when

the mind becomes calm and Prâna has entered the middle channel.

15.) jñānaṃ kuto manasi sambhavatīha tāvat prāṇo|api jīvati mano mriyate na yāvat | prāṇo mano dvayamidaṃ vilayaṃ nayedyo mokṣaṃ sa ghachchati naro na kathaṃchi-danyaḥ

How can it he possible to get knowledge, so long as the Prâna is living and the mind has not died? No one else can get moksa, except one who can make one's Prâna and mind latent.

16.) jñātvā suṣhumṇāsad-bhedaṃ kṛtvā vāyuṃ cha madhyagham | sthitvā sadaiva susthāne brahma-randhre nirodhayet

Always living in a good locality and having known the secret of the Susumnâ, which has a middle course, and making the Vâyu move in it., (the Yogî) should restrain the Vâyu in the Brahma randhra.

17.) sūrya-chandramasau dhattaḥ kālaṃ rātrindivātmakam | bhoktrī suṣhumnā kālasya ghuhyametadudāhṛtam

Time, in the form of night and day, is made by the sun

and the moon. That, the Susumnâ devours this time
(death) even, is a great secret.

18.) dvā-saptati-sahasrāṇi nāḍī-dvārāṇi pañja-re | suṣhumṇā śāmbhavī śaktiḥ śeṣhāstveva nirarthakāḥ

In this body there are 72,000 openings of Nâdis; of these, the Susumnâ, which has the Sâmhhavî Sakti in it, is the only important one, the rest are useless.

19.) vāyuḥ parichito yasmādaghninā saha kuṇḍalīm | bodhayitvā suṣhumṇāyāṃ pra-viśedanirodhataḥ

The Vâyu should be made to enter the Susumnâ without restraint by him who has practised the control of bre-athing and has awakened the Kundali by the (gastric) fire.

20.) suṣhumṇā-vāhini prāṇe siddhyatyeva manonmanī | anyathā tvitarābhyāsāḥ pray-āsāyaiva yoghinām

The Prâna, flowing through the Susumnâ, brings about the condition of manonmanî; other practices are simply futile for the Yogî.

21.) pavano badhyate yena manastenaiva badhyate I manaścha badhyate yena pavanastena badhyate

By whom the breathing has been controlled, by him the activities of the mind also have been controlled; and, conversely, by whom the activities of the mind have been controlled, by him the breathing also has been controlled.

22.) hetu-dvayaṃ tu chittasya vāsanā cha samīraṇaḥ I tayorvinaṣhṭa ekasmintau dvāvapi vinaśyataḥ

There are two causes of the activities of the mind: (1) Vâsanâ (desires) and (2) the respiration (the Prâna). Of these, the destruction of the one is the destruction of both.

23.) mano yatra vilīyeta pavanastatra līyate I pavano līyate yatra manastatra vilīyate

Breathing is lessened when the mind becomes absorbed, and the mind becomes absorbed when the Prâna is restrained.

24.) dughdhāmbuvatsaṃmilitāvubhau tau tulya-kriyau mānasa-mārutau hi | yato maruttatra manaḥ-pravṛttir yato manastatra marut-pravṛttiḥ

Both the mind and the breath are united together, like milk and water; and both of them are equal in their activities. Mind begins its activities where there is the breath, and the Parana begins its activities where there is the mind.

25.) atraika-nāśādaparasya nāśa eka-pravṛt-terapara-pravṛttiḥ | adhvastayośchend-riya-vargha-vṛttiḥ pradhvastayormokṣha-pa-dasya siddhiḥ

By the suspension of the one, therefore, comes the suspension of the other, and by the operations of the one are brought about the operations of the other. When they are present, the Indriyas (the senses) remain engaged in their proper functions, and when they become latent then there is moksa.

26.) rasasya manasaśchaiva chañchalatvaṃ svabhāvataḥ | raso baddho mano baddhaṃ kiṃ na siddhyati bhūtale

By nature, Mercury and mind are unsteady: there is

*nothing in the world which cannot be accomplished
when these are made steady.*

27.) mūrchchito harate vyādhīnmṛto jīvayati svayam | baddhaḥ khecharatām dhatte raso vāyuścha pārvati

*O Pârvati! Mercury and breathing, when made steady,
destroy diseases and the dead himself comes to life (by
their means). By their (proper) control, moving in the
air is attained.*

28.) manaḥ sthairyaṃ sthiro vāyustato binduḥ sthiro bhavet | bindu-sthairyātsadā sattvaṃ piṇḍa-sthairyaṃ prajāyate

*The breathing is calmed when the mind becomes steady
and calm; and hence the preservation of bindu. The
preservation of this latter makes the satwa established in
the body.*

29.) indriyāṇāṃ mano nātho manonāthastu mārutaḥ | mārutasya layo nāthaḥ sa layo nādamāśritaḥ

*Mind is the master of the senses, and the breath is the
master of the mind. The breath in its turn is subordinate*

*to the laya (absorption), and that laya depends on the
nâda.*

30.) so|ayamevāstu mokṣhākhyo māstu vāpi matāntare I manaḥ-prāṇa-laye kaśchidānandaḥ sampravartate

This very laya is what is called moksa, or, being a sectarian, you may not call it moksa; but when the mind becomes absorbed, a sort of ecstacy is experienced.

31.) pranaṣhṭa-śvāsa-niśvāsaḥ pradhvasta-viṣhaya-ghrahaḥ I niścheṣhṭo nirvikāraścha layo jayati yoghinām

By the suspension of respiration and the annihilation of the enjoyments of the senses, when the mind becomes devoid of all the activities and remains changeless, then the Yogî attains to the Laya Stage.

32.) uchchinna-sarva-sangkalp-niḥśeṣhāśeṣha-cheṣhṭitaḥ I svāvaghamyo layaḥ ko|api jāyate vāgh-aghocharaḥ

All the prominent desires being entirely finished, and the body motionless, results in the absorption or laya, which is only known by the Self, and beyond the scope of words.

**33.) yatra dṛṣhṭirlayastatra bhūtend-
riya-sanātanī I sā śaktirjīva-bhūtānāṃ dve
alakṣhye layaṃ ghate**

*Where the sight is directed, absorption occurs. That in
which the elements, senses and shakti exist externally,
which is in all living things, both ore dissolved in the
characteristicless.*

**34.) layo laya iti prāhuḥ kīdṛ́śaṃ laya-
lakṣhaṇam I apunar-vāsanotthānāllayo
viṣhaya-vismṛ́tiḥ**

*Some say 'laya, laya' but what is the characteristic of
laya or absorption? Laya is the non-recollection of the
objects of the senses when the previous deep-rooted
desires (and impressions) are non-recurrent.*

**35.) veda-śāstra-purāṇāni sāmānya-ghaṇikā
iva I ekaiva śāmbhavī mudrā ghuptā ku-
la-vadhūriva**

*The Vedas, shastras and Puranas are like common
women, but shambhavi is secret like a woman of good
heritage.*

36.) atha śāmbhavī

antarlakṣhyaṃ bahirdṛṣhṭirnimeṣhonme-
ṣha-varjitā ǀ eṣhā sā śāmbhavī mudrā ve-
da-śāstreṣhu ghopitā

The Sâmbhavî Mudrâ.

With internalized (one-pointed) awareness and external gaze unblinking, that verily is shambhavi mudra, preserved in the Vedas.

37.) antarlakṣhya-vilīna-chitta-pavano yoghī
yadā vartate dṛṣhṭyā niśchala-tārayā bahirad-
haḥ paśyannapaśyannapi ǀ mudreyaṃ khalu
śāmbhavī bhavati sā labdhā prasādādghuroḥ
śūnyāśūnya-vilakṣhaṇaṃ sphurati tattattvaṃ
padaṃ śāmbhavam

When the Yogî remains inwardly attentive to the Brahman, keeping the mind and the Prâna absorbed, and the sight steady, as if seeing everything while in reality seeing nothing outside, below, or above, verily then it is called the Sâmbhavî Mudrâ, which is learnt by the favour of a guru. Whatever, wonderful, Sûnya or Asûnya is perceived, is to be regarded as the manifestation of that great Śambhû (Śiva.)

**38.) śrī-śāmbhavyāścha khecharyā avast-
hā-dhāma-bhedataḥ | bhavechchitta-layā-
nandaḥ śūnye chit-sukha-rūpiṇi**

*The two states, the Sâmbhavî and the Khecharî, are
different because of their seats (being the heart and
the space between the eyebrows respectively); but both
cause happiness, for the mind becomes absorbed in the
Chita-sukha-Rupa-âtmana which is void.*

**39.) tāre jyotiṣhi saṃyojya kiṃchidunnamay-
edbhruvau | pūrva-yoghaṃ mano yuñjan-
nunmanī-kārakaḥ kṣhaṇāt**

*With perfect concentration, the pupils fixed on the light
by raising the eyebrows up a little, as from the previously described (shambhavi), mind is joined and instantly
unmani occurs.*

**40.) kechidāghama-jālena kechinnigha-
ma-sangkulaiḥ | kechittarkeṇa muhyanti
naiva jānanti tārakam**

*Some are devoted to the Vedas, some to Nigama, while
others are enwrapt in Logic, but none knows the value
of this mudrâ, which enables one to cross the ocean of
existence.*

41.) ardhonmīlita-lochanaḥ sthira-manā nāsāghra-dattekṣhaṇaś chandrārkāvapi lī-natāmupanayannispanda-bhāvena yaḥ । jyo-tī-rūpamaśeṣha-bījamakhilaṃ dedīpyamānaṃ paraṃ tattvaṃ tat-padameti vastu paramaṃ vāchyaṃ kimatrādhikam

With steady calm mind and half closed eyes, fixed on the tip of the nose, stopping the Idâ and the Pingalâ without blinking, he who can see the light which is the all, the seed, the entire brilliant, great Tatwama, app-roaches Him, who is the great object. What is the use of more talk?

42.) divā na pūjayellingghaṃ rātrau chai-va na pūjayet । sarvadā pūjayellingghaṃ divārātri-nirodhataḥ

One should not meditate on the Linga (i.e., Âtman) in the day (i.e., while Sûrya or Pingalâ is working) or at night (when Idâ is working), but should always cont-emplate after restraining both.

43.) atha khecharī savya-dakṣhiṇa-nāḍī-stho madhye cha-rati mārutaḥ । tiṣhṭhate khecharī mudrā tasminsthāne na saṃśayaḥ

The Khecharî.

*When the prana which is in the right and left nadis mo-
ves m the middle nadi (sushumna) that is the condition
for khechari mudra.*

44.) iḍā-pingghalayormadhye śūnyaṃ chaivā-
nilaṃ ghraset | tiṣhṭhate khecharī mudrā
tatra satyaṃ punaḥ punaḥ

*The fire (of shakti) being swallowed (suppressed) mid-
way between, ida and pingala, in that shoonya (of sushumna), is in truth the condition for khechari mudra.*

45.) sūrchyāchandramasormadhye nirālam-
bāntare punaḥ | saṃsthitā vyoma-chakre yā
sā mudrā nāma khecharī

*That Mudrâ is called Khecharî which is performed in
the supportless space between the Sûrya and the Chandra (the Idâ and the Pingalâ) and called the Vyoma
Chakra.*

46.) somādyatroditā dhārā sākṣhātsā śiva-val-
labhā | pūrayedatulāṃ divyāṃ suṣhumṇāṃ
paśchime mukhe

*The Khecharî which causes the stream to flow from the
Chandra (Śoma) is beloved of Śiva. The incomparable
divine Susumnâ should be closed by the tongue drawn
back.*

47.) purastāchchaiva pūryeta niśchitā khecharī bhavet I abhyastā khecharī mud-rāpyunmanī samprajāyate

*It can be closed from the front also (by stopping the mo-
vements of the Prâna), and then surely it becomes the
Khecharî. By practice, this Khecharî leads to Unmanî.*

48.) bhruvormadhye śiva-sthānaṃ manastatra vilīyate I jñātavyaṃ tat-padaṃ turyaṃ tatra kālo na vidyate

*In the middle of the Eyebrows is the place of Shiva, there
the mind is quiescent. That state is known as turiya or
the fourth dimension. There, time is unknown.*

49.) abhyasetkhecharīṃ tāvadyāvatsyādyog-ha-nidritaḥ I samprāpta-yogha-nidrasya kālo nāsti kadāchana

*The Khecharî should be practised till there is Yoga-nidrâ
(Samâdhi). One who has induced Yoga-nidrâ, cannot
fall a victim to death.*

**50.) nirālambaṃ manaḥ kṛtvā na kiṃchida-
pi chintayet | sa-bāhyābhyantaraṃ vyomni
ghaṭavattiṣhṭhati dhruvam**

*Freeing the mind from all thoughts and thinking of
nothing, one should sit firmly like a pot in the space
(surrounded and filled with the ether).*

**51.) bāhya-vāyuryathā līnastathā madhyo na
saṃśayaḥ | sva-sthāne sthiratāmeti pavano
manasā saha**

*As the air, in and out of the body, remains unmoved, so
the breath with mind becomes steady in its place (i.e., in
Brahma randhra).*

**52.) evamabhyasyatastasya vāyu-mārghe
divāniśam | abhyāsājjīryate vāyurmanasta-
traiva līyate**

*By thus practising, night and day, the breathing is
brought under control, and, as the practice increases, the
mind becomes calm and steady.*

**53.) amṛtaiḥ plāvayeddehamāpāda-tala-mas-
takam | siddhyatyeva mahā-kāyo mahā-ba-
la-parākramaḥ**

*By rubbing the body over with Amrita (exuding from
the moon), from head to foot, one gets Mahâkâyâ, i.e.,
great strength and energy.*

End of the Khecharî.

54.) śakti-madhye manaḥ kṛtvā śaktiṃ mā-
nasa-madhyaghām | manasā mana ālokya
dhārayetparamaṃ padam

*Placing the mind into the Kundalini, and getting the
latter into the mind, by looking upon the Buddhi (intellect) with mind (reflexively), the Param Pada (Brahma)
should be obtained.*

55.) kha-madhye kuru chātmānamātma-mad-
hye cha khaṃ kuru | sarvaṃ cha kha-mayaṃ
kṛtvā na kiṃchidapi chintayet

*Keep the âtmâ inside the Kha (Brahma) and place
Brahma inside your âtmâ. Having made everything
pervaded with Kha (Brahma), think of nothing else.*

56.) antaḥ śūnyo bahiḥ śūnyaḥ śūnyaḥ kum-
bha ivāmbare | antaḥ pūrṇo bahiḥ pūrṇaḥ
pūrṇaḥ kumbha ivārṇave

One should become void in and void out, and voice like

*a pot in the space. Full in and full outside, like a jar in
the ocean.*

57.) bāhya-chintā na kartavyā tathaivānta-ra-chintanam | sarva-chintāṃ parityajya na kiṃchidapi chintayet

*He should be neither of his inside nor of outside world;
and, leaving all thoughts, he should think of nothing.*

58.) sangkalpa-mātra-kalanaiva jaghatsam-aghraṃ sangkalpa-mātra-kalanaiva ma-no-vilāsaḥ | sangkalpa-mātra-matimutsṛja nirvikalpam āśritya niśchayamavāpnuhi rāma śāntim

*The whole of this world and all the schemes of the
mind are but the creations of thought. Discarding these
thoughts and taking leave of all conjectures, O Râma!
obtain peace.*

59.) karpūramanale yadvatsaindhavaṃ salile yathā | tathā sandhīyamānaṃ cha manas-tattve vilīyate

*As camphor disappears in fire, and rock salt in water, so
the mind united with the âtmâ loses its identity.*

**60.) jñeyaṃ sarvaṃ pratītaṃ cha jñānaṃ
cha mana uchyate | jñānaṃ jñeyaṃ samaṃ
naṣhṭaṃ nānyaḥ panthā dvitīyakaḥ**

*When the knowable, and the knowledge, are both
destroyed equally, then there is no second way (i.e.,
Duality is destroyed).*

**61.) mano-dṛśyamidaṃ sarvaṃ yat-
kiṃchitsa-charācharam | manaso hyun-
manī-bhāvāddvaitaṃ naivolabhyate**

*All this movable and immovable world is mind. When
the mind has attained to the unmanî avasthâ, there
is no dwaita (from the absence of the working of the
mind.)*

**62.) jñeya-vastu-parityāghādvilayaṃ yāti
mānasam | manaso vilaye jāte kaivalyama-
vaśiṣhyate**

*Mind disappears by removing the knowable, and, on its
disappearance, âtmâ only remains behind.*

**63.) evaṃ nānā-vidhopāyāḥ samy-
aksvānubhavānvitāḥ | samādhi-mārghāḥ
kathitāḥ pūrvāchāryairmahātmabhiḥ**

The high-souled Âchâryas (Teachers) of yore gained experience in the various methods of Samâdhi themselves, and then they preached them to others.

64.) suṣhumṇāyai kuṇḍalinyai sudhāyai ch-andra-janmane | manonmanyai namastubhy-aṃ mahā-śaktyai chid-ātmane

Salutations to Thee, O Susumnâ, to Thee O Kundalinî, to Thee O Sudhâ, born of Chandra, to Thee O Manom-nanî! to Thee O great power, energy and the intelligent spirit.

65.) aśakya-tattva-bodhānāṃ mūḍhānāmapi sammatam | proktaṃ ghorakṣha-nāthena nādopāsanamuchyate

I will describe now the practice of anâhata nâda, as propounded by Goraksa Nâtha, for the benefit of those who are unable to understand the principles of knowledge—a method, which is liked by the ignorant also.

66.) śrī-ādināthena sa-pāda-koṭi-laya-prakārāḥ kathitā jayanti | nādānusandhānakamekame-va manyāmahe mukhyatamaṃ layānām

Âdinâtha propounded 1¼ crore methods of trance, and

*they are all extant. Of these, the hearing of the anâhata
nâda is the Only one, the chief, in my opinion.*

67.) muktāsane sthito yoghī mudrāṃ sand-
hāya śāmbhavīm | śṛṇuyāddakṣhiṇe karṇe
nādamantāsthamekadhīḥ

*Sitting with Mukta Âsana and with the Sâmbhavî Ma-
dill, the Yogî should hear the sound inside his right ear,
with collected mind.*

68.) śravaṇa-puṭa-nayana-yughala
ghrāṇa-mukhānāṃ nirodhanaṃ kāryam |
śuddha-suṣhumṇā-saraṇau sphuṭamamalaḥ
śrūyate nādaḥ

*The ears, the eyes, the nose, and the mouth should be
closed and then the clear sound is heard in the passage of the Susumnâ which has been cleansed of all its
impurities.*

69.) ārambhaścha ghaṭaśchaiva tathā pa-
richayo|api cha | niṣhpattiḥ sarva-yogheṣhu
syādavasthā-chatuṣhṭayam

*In all the Yogas, there are four states: (1) ârambha or the
preliminary, (2) Ghata, or the state of a jar, (3) Parichaya (known), (4) nispatti (consumate.)*

70.) atha ārambhāvasthā
brahma-ghrantherbhavedbhedo hyānandaḥ
śūnya-sambhavaḥ | vichitraḥ kvaṇako de-
he|anāhataḥ śrūyate dhvaniḥ

Ârambha Avasthâ.

When the Brahma granthi (in the heart) is pierced through by Prânâyâma, then a sort of happiness is experienced in the vacuum of the heart, and the anâhat sounds, like various tinkling sounds of ornaments, are heard in the body.

71.) divya-dehaścha tejasvī divya-ghandhas-
tvaroghavān | sampūrṇa-hṛdayaḥ śūnya
ārambhe yoghavānbhavet

In the ârambha, a Yogî's body becomes divine, glowing, healthy, and emits a divine swell. The whole of his heart becomes void.

72.) atha ghaṭāvasthā
dvitīyāyāṃ ghaṭīkṛtya vāyurbhavati mad-
hyaghaḥ | dṛḍhāsano bhavedyoghī jñānī
deva-samastadā

The Ghata Avasthâ.

In the second stage, the airs are united into one and begin moving in the middle channel. The Yogî's posture becomes firm, and he becomes wise like a god.

73.) viṣhṇu-ghranthestato bhedātparamā-nanda-sūchakaḥ I atiśūnye vimardaścha bherī-śabdastadā bhavet

By this means the Vishu knot (in the throat) is pierced which is indicated by highest pleasure experienced, And then the Bherî sound (like the beating of a kettle drain) is evolved in the vacuum in the throat.

74.) atha parichayāvasthā tṛtīyāyāṃ tu vijñeyo vihāyo mardala-dhva-niḥ I mahā-śūnyaṃ tadā yāti sarva-sidd-hi-samāśrayam

The Parichaya Avasthâ.

In the third stage, the sound of a drum is known to arise in tie Sûnya between the eyebrows, and then the Vâyu goes to the Mahâśûnya, which is the home of all the siddhîs.

75.) chittānandaṃ tadā jitvā sahajānan-

**da-sambhavaḥ | doṣa-duḥkha-jarā-vyād-
hi-kṣhudhā-nidrā-vivarjitaḥ**

*Conquering, then, the pleasures of the mind, ecstacy is
spontaneously produced which is devoid of evils, pains,
old age, disease, hunger and sleep.*

**76.) atha niṣhpatty-avasthā
rudra-ghranthiṃ yadā bhittvā śar-
va-pīṭha-ghato|anilaḥ | niṣhpattau vaiṇavaḥ
śabdaḥ kvaṇad-vīṇā-kvaṇo bhavet**

The Nishpatty Avasthâ.

*When the Rudra granthi is pierced and the air enters the
seat of the Lord (the space between the eyebrows), then
the perfect sound like that of a flute is produced.*

**77.) ekībhūtaṃ tadā chittaṃ rāja-yoghābhid-
hānakam | sṛṣhṭi-saṃhāra-kartāsau yog-
hīśvara-samo bhavet**

*The union of the mind and the sound is called the
Râja-Yoga. The (real) Yogî becomes the creator and
destroyer of the universe, like God.*

78.) astu vā māstu vā muktiratraivākhaṇḍi-

tam sukham | layodbhavamidam saukhyam rāja-yoghādavāpyate

Perpetual Happiness is achieved by this; I do not care if the mukti be not attained. This happiness, resulting from absorption [in Brahma], is obtained by means of Raja-Yoga.

79.) rāja-yoghamajānantaḥ kevalam haṭha-karmiṇaḥ | etānabhyāsino manye prayāsa-phala-varjitān

Those who are ignorant of the Râja-Yoga and practise only the Hatha-Yoga, will, in my opinion, waste their energy fruitlessly.

80.) unmany-avāptaye śīghram bhrū-dhyā-nam mama sammatam | rāja-yogha-padam prāptum sukhopāyo|alpa-chetasām | sadyaḥ pratyaya-sandhāyī jāyate nādajo layaḥ

Contemplation on the space between the eyebrows is, in my opinion, best for accomplishing soon the Unmanî state. For people of small intellect, it is a very easy method for obtaining perfection in the Raja-Yoga. The Laya produced by nâda, at once gives experience (of spiritual powers).

**81.) nādānusandhāna-samādhi-bhājāṃ yog-
hīśvarāṇāṃ hṛdi vardhamānam l ānandame-
kaṃ vachasāmaghamyaṃ jānāti taṃ śrī-ghu-
runātha ekaḥ**

*The happiness which increases in the hearts of Yogiśwa-
ras, who have gained success in Samâdhi by means of
attention to the nâda, is beyond description, and is
known to Śri Gurû Nâtha alone.*

**82.) karṇau pidhāya hastābhyāṃ yaḥ śṛṇoti
dhvaniṃ muniḥ l tatra chittaṃ sthirīkuryā-
dyāvatsthira-padaṃ vrajet**

*The sound which a muni hears by closing his ears with
his fingers, should be heard attentively, till the mind
becomes steady in it.*

**83.) abhyasyamāno nādo|ayaṃ bāhyamāvṛṇu-
te dhvanim l pakṣhādvikṣhepamakhilaṃ
jitvā yoghī sukhī bhavet**

*By practising with this nâda, all other external sounds
are stopped. The Yogî becomes happy by overcoming all
distractions within 15 days.*

**84.) śrūyate prathamābhyāse nādo nānā-vid-
ho mahān | tato|abhyāse vardhamāne śrūya-
te sūkṣhma-sūkṣhmakaḥ**

*In the beginning, the sounds heard are of great variety
and very loud; but, as the practice increases, they become more and more subtle.*

**85.) ādau jaladhi-jīmūta-bherī-jharjhara-sam-
bhavāḥ | madhye mardala-śangkhotthā
ghaṇṭā-kāhalajāstathā**

*In the first stage, the sounds are surging, thundering like
the beating of kettle drums and jingling ones. In the intermediate stage, they are like those produced by conch,
Mridanga, bells, &c.*

**86.) ante tu kingkiṇī-vaṃśa-vīṇā-bhramara-
niḥsvanāḥ | iti nānāvidhā nādāḥ śrūyante
deha-madhyaghāḥ**

*In the last stage, the sounds resemble those from tinklets,
flute, bee, &c. These various kinds of sounds are heard
as being produced in the body.*

**87.) mahati śrūyamāṇe|api megha-bhery-ādi-
ke dhvanau | tatra sūkṣhmātsūkṣhmataraṃ
nādameva parāmṛśet**

Though hearing loud sounds like those of thunder, kettle drums, etc. one should practise with the subtle sounds also.

88.) ghanamutsṝjya vā sūkṣhme sūkṣhmamutsṝjya vā ghane ǀ ramamāṇamapi kṣhiptaṃ mano nānyatra chālayet

Leaving the loudest, taking up the subtle one, and leaving the subtle one, taking up the loudest, thus practising, the distracted mind does not wander elsewhere.

89.) yatra kutrāpi vā nāde laghati prathamaṃ manaḥ ǀ tatraiva susthirībhūya tena sārdhaṃ vilīyate

Wherever the mind attaches itself first, it becomes steady there; and then it becomes absorbed in it.

90.) makarandaṃ pibanbhṝṅgghī ghandhaṃ nāpekṣhate yathā ǀ nādāsaktaṃ tathā chittaṃ viṣhayānnahi kāṅgkṣhate

Just as a bee, drinking sweet juice, does not care for the smell of the flower; so the mind, absorbed in the nâda, does not desire the objects of enjoyment.

**91.) mano-matta-ghajendrasya viṣhayodyā-
na-chāriṇaḥ | samartho|ayaṃ niyamane
nināda-niśitāngkuśaḥ**

*The mind, like an elephant habituated to wander in the
garden of enjoyments, is capable of being controlled by
the sharp goad of anâhata nâda.*

**92.) baddhaṃ tu nāda-bandhena manaḥ san-
tyakta-chāpalam | prayāti sutarāṃ sthairyaṃ
chinna-pakṣhaḥ khagho yathā**

*The mind, captivated in the snare of nâda, gives up all
its activity; and, like a bird with clipped wings, becomes
calm at once.*

**93.) sarva-chintāṃ parityajya sāvadhānena
chetasā | nāda evānusandheyo yogha-sām-
rājyamichchhatā**

*Those desirous of the kingdom of Yoga, should take up
the practice of hearing the anâhata nâda, with mind
collected and free from all cares.*

**94.) nādo|antaranggha-sāranggha-bandhane
vāghurāyate | antaranggha-kurangghasya
vadhe vyādhāyate|api cha**

Nada is the snare for catching the mind; and, when it is caught like a deer, it can be killed also like it.

95.) antarangghasya yamino vājinaḥ parig-hāyate I nādopāsti-rato nityamavadhāryā hi yoghinā

Nâda is the bolt of the stable door for the horse (the minds of the Yogîs). A Yogî should determine to practise constantly in the hearing of the nâda sounds.

96.) baddhaṃ vimukta-chāñchalyaṃ nā-da-ghandhaka-jāraṇāt I manaḥ-pāradamāp-noti nirālambākhya-khe|aṭanam

Mind gets the properties of calcined mercury. When deprived of its unsteadiness it is calcined, combined with the sulphur of nâda, and then it roams like it in tine supportless âkâśa or Brahma. 95.

97.) nāda-śravaṇataḥ kṣhipramantarangg-ha-bhujangghamam I vismṛtaya sarva-mekāghraḥ kutrachinnahi dhāvati

The mind is like a serpent, forgetting all its unsteadiness by hearing the nâda, it does not run away anywhere.

**98.) kāṣṭhe pravartito vahniḥ kāṣṭhena
saha śāmyati I nāde pravartitaṃ chittaṃ
nādena saha līyate**

*The fire, catching firewood, is extinguished along with
it (after burning it up); and so the mind also, working
with the nâda, becomes latent along with it.*

**99.) ghaṇṭādināda-sakta-stabdhāntaḥ-ka-
raṇa-hariṇasya I praharaṇamapi sukaraṃ
syāchchara-sandhāna-pravīṇaśchet**

*The antahkarana (mind), like a deer, becomes absorbed
and motionless on hearing the sound of hells, etc. and
then it is very easy for an expert archer to kill it.*

**100.) anāhatasya śabdasya dhvanirya upa-
labhyate I dhvanerantarghataṃ jñeyaṃ jñey-
asyāntarghataṃ manaḥ I manastatra layaṃ
yāti tadviṣhṇoḥ paramaṃ padam**

*The knowable interpenetrates the anâhata sound which
is heard, and the mind interpenetrates the knowable.
The mind becomes absorbed there, which is the seat of
the all-pervading, almighty Lord.*

101.) tāvadākāśa-sangkalpo yāvachchabdaḥ pravartate | niḥśabdaṃ tat-paraṃ brahma paramāteti ghīyate

So long as the sounds continue, there is the idea of âkâśa. When they disappear, then it is called Para Brahma, Paramâtmana.

102.) yatkiṃchinnāda-rūpeṇa śrūyate śaktire-va sā | yastattvānto nirākāraḥ sa eva para-meśvaraḥ

Whatever is heard in the form of nâda, is the śakti (power). That which is formless, the final state of the Tatwas, is tile Parameśwara.

103.) iti nādānusandhānam sarve haṭha-layopāyā rājayoghasya sidd-haye | rāja-yogha-samārūḍhaḥ puruṣhaḥ kāla-vañchakaḥ

All the methods of Hatha are meant for gaining success in the Raja-Yoga; for, the man, who is well-established in the Raja-Yoga, overcomes death.

104.) tattvam bījam haṭhaḥ kṣhetra-maudāsīnyam jalam tribhiḥ | unmanī kal-pa-latikā sadya eva pravartate

*Tatwa is the seed, Hatha the field; and Indifference
(Vairâgya) the water. By the action of these three, the
creeper Unmanî thrives very rapidly.*

105.) sadā nādānusandhānātkṣhīyante pā-pa-saṃchayāḥ I nirañjane vilīyete niśchitaṃ chitta-mārutau

*All the accumulations of sins are destroyed by practising
always with the nâda; and the mind and the airs do
certainly become latent in the colorless (Paramâtmana).*

106.) śangkha-dundhubhi-nādaṃ cha na śṝṇoti kadāchana I kāṣhṭhavajjāyate deha unmanyāvasthayā dhruvam

*Such a one. does not hear the noise of the conch and
Dundubhi. Being in the Unmanî avasthâ, his body becomes like a piece of wood.*

107.) sarvāvasthā-vinirmuktaḥ sar-va-chintā-vivarjitaḥ I mṛtavattiṣhṭhate yoghī sa mukto nātra saṃśayaḥ

*There is no doubt, such a Yogî becomes free from all
states, from all cares, and remains like one dead.*

**108.) khādyate na cha kālena bādhyate na
cha karmaṇā | sādhyate na sa kenāpi yoghī
yuktaḥ samādhinā**

*He is not devoured by death, is not bound by his
actions. The Yogî who is engaged in Samâdhi is over-
powered by none.*

**109.) na ghandhaṃ na rasaṃ rūpaṃ na cha
sparśaṃ na niḥsvanam | nātmānaṃ na pa-
raṃ vetti yoghī yuktaḥ samādhinā**

*The Yogî, engaged in Samâdhi, feels neither smell, taste,
color, touch, sound, nor is conscious of his own self.*

**110.) chittaṃ na suptaṃ nojāghratsmṛ-
ti-vismṛti-varjitam | na chāstameti nodeti
yasyāsau mukta eva saḥ**

*He whose mind is neither sleeping, waking, remembe-
ring, destitute of memory, disappearing nor appearing,
is liberated.*

**111.) na vijānāti śītoṣhṇaṃ na duḥkhaṃ na
sukhaṃ tathā | na mānaṃ nopamānaṃ cha
yoghī yuktaḥ samādhinā**

He feels neither heat, cold, pain, pleasure, respect nor disrespect. Such a Yogî is absorbed in Samâdhi.

112.) svastho jāghradavasthāyāṃ suptava-dyo|avatiṣhṭhate | niḥśvāsochchvāsa-hī-naścha niśchitaṃ mukta eva saḥ

He who, though awake, appears like one sleeping, and is without inspiration and expiration, is certainly free.

113.) avadhyaḥ sarva-śastrāṇāmaśakyaḥ sarva-dehinām | aghrāhyo mantra-yantrāṇāṃ yoghī yuktaḥ samādhinā

The Yogî, engaged in Samâdhi, cannot be killed by any instrument, and is beyond the controlling power of beings. He is beyond the reach of incantations and charms.

114.) yāvadvidurna bhavati dṛḍhaḥ prāṇa-vāta-prabandhāt | yāvaddhyāne saha-ja-sadṛśaṃ jāyate naiva tattvaṃ tāvajjñānaṃ vadati tadidaṃ dambha-mithyā-pralāpaḥ

As long as the Prâna does not enter and flow in the middle channel and the vindu does not become firm by the control of the movements of the Prâna; as long as the mind does not assume the form of Brahma without any

effort in contemplation, so long all the talk of knowledge
and wisdom is merely the nonsensical babbling of a mad
man.

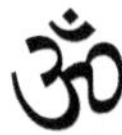

iti haṭha-yogha-pradīpikāyāṃ samād-
hi-lakṣhaṇaṃ nāma chaturthopadeśaḥ |

THE END.

KUNDALINI YOGA

ALL ABOUT OUR CHAKRA!

BESTSELLING AUTHOR

Shreyananda Natha

NAMASTÉ

I want to thank the teachers and students I have had over the years and who have made my journey with yoga so interesting. Thank you for all the inspiration you have given me and for making this book possible. The yoga masters who no longer live among us, live on with every new person who immerses themselves in the yoga tradition.

Sri Swami Sivananda, Sri Swami Satyananda, Sri Tirumalai Krishnamacharya, Sri Swami Vishnudevananda, Sri K. Pattabhi Jois, Osho, Swami Nirdosha, Swami Omananda, Swami Janakananda, Ole Schmidt, Turiya, Maryam Abrishami and Sanna Kuittinen.

Everyone who has searched for answers to what they perceived through an activated ajna chakra. In yoga, they have learned the principles behind the universe, the collective consciousness, and the creative power, Kundalini Shakti. The duality behind everything, both what we see and what we do not see. Together we help to pass on the previous secret knowledge, about our gunas, nadis, and chakras, to anyone who wants to be seen.

THE AUTHOR

Shreyananda Natha is the author of over twelve titles on yoga. Among other things, he has written the most comprehensive books on yoga in Swedish – Everything About Yoga and the study book The Yoga Bible. He is also a certified yoga and meditation teacher according to EYTF's international guidelines and has undergone a multi-year yoga teacher training under the leadership of Swami Omananda at Satyananda Ashram. Shreyananda Natha holds the highest initiation in the Tantric Natha Order. He travels frequently to Asia and India to improve himself, and to gain knowledge and inspiration. He has immersed himself in the tantric rituals and is known for his extensive knowledge of yoga, deep relaxation, and meditation

There is no authority that can say what yoga is. When you give yourself fully and completely, and experience yoga without limitations or doubts, when you become one with the true experience in yourself, the real encounter with yoga arises. Only then do you understand what yoga is – for you. You are no longer limited by ornament, shyness and artificial thought patterns that lie as a filter between you and the transformation. Yoga is a cultural-historical wealth that is still passed on from teacher to student and helps man to find his way back to his true nature. It opens us up and attracts awareness.

It strengthens our self-esteem, and our entire person's spectrum of possibilities suddenly becomes visible to us. Yoga is not difficult. You do not have to be vegan or able to stand on your head. You just need to practice your yoga regularly and the rest will come by itself.

With all the love from the universe – Aum Shanti Shreyananda Natha.

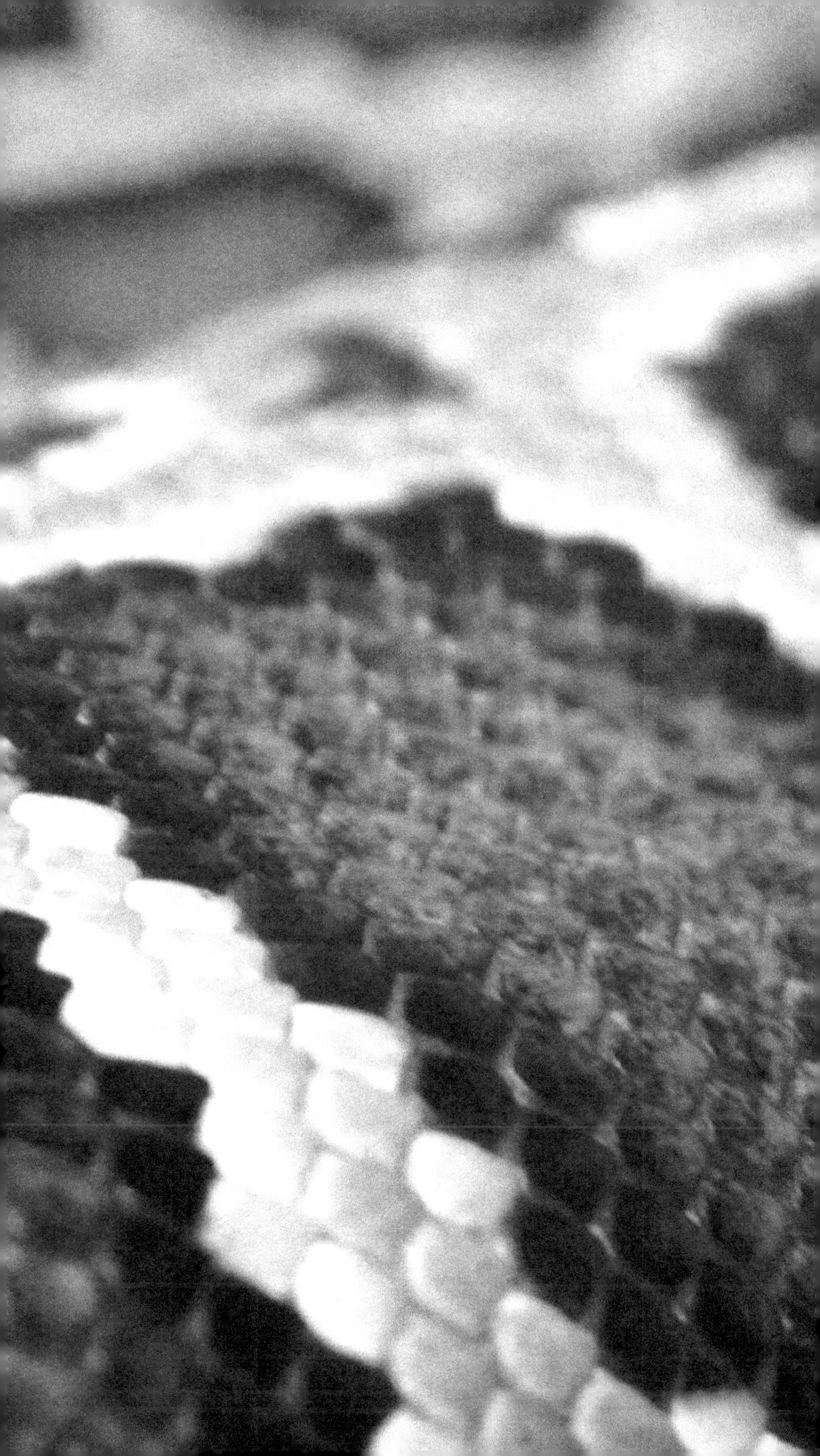

KUNDALINI YOGA

WHAT IS KUNDALINI?

Kundalini is what we call the dormant energy that exists in every human being. It has its seat at the bottom of the spine in the perineum, or pelvic floor, (between the urine and the excretory organs) in men and at the cervix (the bottom of the cervix in women). This is also where the Mooladhara chakra is found.

With the help of yogic techniques such as asana, pranayama, Kriya yoga and meditation, one can increase the flow of prana in the body and direct it down to Mooladhara in order to awaken the Kundalini shakti. When the Kundalini energy then begins to rise upwards along the Sushumna nadi and through the chakras, the dormant parts of the brain that are in contact with the respective chakras are awakened. Through this process, we can have greater access to the capacity of our brain and raise our consciousness.

Awakening of Kundalini should be done slowly and systematically. The body and mind should be prepared slowly. This way, you avoid any risks that a rise may entail. One should not try to control or influence the mind as such. The mind is an "extension" of the body and therefore it is easiest to start with the body and gradually move on with prana, nadis and chakras.

HOW THE KUNDALINI WAS DISCOVERED

Since the beginning, man has been involved in, and experienced events of a supernatural nature. When it so happened that one would feel what others were thinking and wanting, the inner visions manifested and dreams came true. It was noticed that a certain crowd of people had a very special ability to express their creativity through art, music and poetry. Some people had a strong drive, zest for life while others barely managed to get up in the morning. Man became curious as to what was the cause of these differences. In the end, through one's own experience, one could come to the conclusion that in man there was a special form of energy. In some, this energy was dormant, in development in others, and fully awakened in very few. This energy was called after gods and deities. After they also discovered prana, they started calling it prana shakti. In Tantrism, this energy is called Kundalini shakti.

DIFFERENT NAMES

In Sanskrit, Kundalini means "spiral" or "something that is rolled up". Kundalini shakti has thus traditionally been described as something that has just been rolled up. Nevertheless, the meaning of the whole thing has often

been misunderstood. Kundalini actually derives from
the word - kunda, which refers to "a deeper place", or a
pit. The place where a dead body is burned is also called
a customer. The word Kundalini refers to Shakti, or the
power, energy in its dormant state. When it then wakes
up and manifests itself, it is called Devi, Kali, Durga,
Saraswati, Lakshmi or something else depending on the
characteristics and qualities that it evokes in man.

In Christianity, terms such as "the path of the initi-
ated" or "the stairs to heaven" are used. These refer
to the Kundalini that rise along the sushumna. The
Christian cross symbolizes Kundalini rising and the
resulting spiritual beauty. In all spiritual paths, whether
one is talking about samadhi, nirvana, moksha, unity,
kaivalya or liberation, it is Kundalini awakening one is
referring to.

KUNDALINI, DURGA, KALI

When you can handle a raised Kundalini in a positive
way, its quality is called Durga. If Kundalini instead
wakes up when you are still unprepared and not ready
to handle it, it is called Kali.

The goddess Kali is illustrated as naked, black in color
and she wears a rosary of one hundred and eight human
skulls that represent memories from previous lives. Her

*blood-red outstretched tongue symbolizes rajo guna
whose circular movement pattern gives power to all creative activity. She wants to urge sadhakas to take control
of rajo guna.*

*Durga is a beautiful goddess who is illustrated riding
a tiger. She has eight arms that represent the eightfold
elements. She wears a rosary with fifty-two human
skulls that symbolize her wisdom, power and the fifty-
two letters of the Sanskrit alphabet. Durga eliminates
all the evil consequences that life can carry with it, and
comes with power and peace. This force is released from
Mooladhara.*

KUNDALINI PHYSIOLOGY

*When Kundalini begins to rise, it passes different phases
on its way up to the cosmic consciousness - Shiva, where
they finally merge. The highest consciousness - Shiva,
has its seat in Sahasrara - the super consciousness,
at the top of the head. In the Vedic texts as well as in
Tantrism, this seat is called Hiranyagarbha - the womb
of consciousness. It is connected to the pituitary gland.
Just below there is another psychic center called the Ajna
chakra which is connected to the pineal gland, the seat
of intuitive consciousness. It is located at the top of the
spine and at the height of the eyebrow center - bhrumadhya. Ajna chakra is important as it is connected to
both Mooladhara and Sahasrara chakra.*

Chakras are energy vortices that are experienced to vibrate and rotate at different speeds. There are thousands of chakras in the human body. In tantra and yoga, only a few are used for filling the entire spectrum of human evolution and life - physically and mentally, from the rough to the polished. There are six chakras that have a direct connection to the dormant parts of the brain.

Through nadis, energy flows to and from the chakras. Nadis are channels where prana (vital) and mana (mental) energy flows through and out to all parts of the body. There are about seventy-two thousand nadis. Three of these are extra important as they control the flow of prana and the consciousness of all other nadis. These are ida, pingala and sushumna. Ida controls all the mental activity and pingala all the vital activity. Ida is known as the moon and pingala as the sun. Sushumna is the channel for the flow of spiritual consciousness. Ida and pingala do not flow in the body at the same time but they alternate. When the left nostril is open, ida nadi flows and when the right nostril is open, the pingala flows. When the pingala flows, the left part of the brain is active and when the ida flows, the right part of the brain is active. In this way, nadis control our brain, way of acting and consciousness.

If you can get prana and chitta, ie. ida and pingala flow

at the same time, you can also get both halves of the brain to cooperate in thinking and action. This does not happen in our normal daily lives. For this to happen, it is required that the sushi humna is in contact with Kundalini shakti.

Sushumna nadi is like a hollow tube with three more tubes in it. One is more subtle than the other. These tubes, or nadis, are called sushumna (denotes tamas), vajrini (denotes rajas), chitrini (denotes sattva) and Brahma (denotes consciousness). The highest consciousness born of Kundalini shakti passes through Brahma.

When Kundalini wakes up, the sushumna passes up to the Ajna chakra. Mooladhara acts as a powerful engine. To start this engine, pranic energy is needed and it is created with the help of pranayamas. The prana is then directed downwards in the body, to the Mooladhara chakra. From there it is then directed upwards towards the Ajna chakra. If the sushumna nadi is not open, the energy cannot be distributed, which means that the prana remains in the Mooladhara chakra.

Ida and pingala nadi are constantly flowing but their power is weak. It is only when the sushumna is awakened that enlightenment can take place. Kundalini yoga is based on awakening the sushumna, and when awakened, the contact between the highest and lowest levels of

*consciousness is enabled. Then Kundalini can wake up
and rise from Mooladhara up along the sushumna and
then become one with Shiva in Sahasrara.*

THE MYSTICAL TREE

*In Bhagavad Gita you can read about the immortal
tree that grows up and down, with the roots up and the
leaves and branches down. It is said that he who knows
the tree also knows the truth of life. This tree is found in
the human body and nervous system. Thoughts, feelings,
obstacles, etc. symbolized by the leaves of the tree. The
brain is symbolized by the roots and the spine of the
trunk. You have to climb from the top of the tree (in
this case from the root) and up to the roots. In Kabba-
lah, this tree is called the "tree of life". In the Bible it is
called the "tree of knowledge." Anyone who tries to move
upwards from Mooladhara to Sahasrara thus climbs to
the roots.*

KUNDALINI AND OUR BRAIN

*Humans are often said to use only a tenth of the full
capacity of the brain. The knowledge we have, what
we think and do is stored in this small part. The rest is
known as the dormant and inactive part of the brain.
The reason it is inactive is that the amount of energy is
not enough to keep it awake. The active part of the brain
gets its energy from ida and pingala nadi while the dor-*

mant part only has access to pingala ie. prana, or, life energy. It lacks conscious energy, ie. ida, or, manas.

To awaken the sleeping part of the brain, we must charge the front part of the brain with prana and consciousness. We must also awaken sushumna nadi. We do this by practicing pranayamas regularly for an extended period of time. With the help of Kundalini yoga, one could discover that the different parts of the brain were connected to our chakras. To access dormant parts of the brain, one must work on awakening the chakras in the body. Chakras can be described as switches.

The same way, the Mooladhara chakra is used as a "switch" to awaken Kundalini, which actually has its seat in Sahasrara, but most of us find it easier to get in touch with Mooladhara. Each chakra works individually. This means that if Kundalini wakes up in Mooladhara, it goes straight from there up to Sahasrara. Or, if it wakes up in Swadhisthana, it also goes from there straight up to Sahasrara. Kundalini can be awakened in a chakra or collectively in all chakras at the same time. When Kundalini awakens in an individual chakra, the consciousness is filled with what is characteristic of that particular chakra.

WHAT KUNDALINI SHAKTI REALLY IS

There are many different descriptions of what Kundalini shakti really is. Many yogis believe that Kundalini shakti is pranic energy that flows through the sushumna associated with the spine. They believe that Kundalini is part of the pranic flow in our energy body and that there is no physical / anatomical equivalent.

Other yogis experience Kundalini as part of the signals that flow along the nerve pathways and that travel along the spinal cord up to specific parts of the brain. However, most agree that the experience of Kundalini is something psychophysiological that is manifested in the spine.

METHODS FOR AWAKENING:

In Tantrism, various techniques are used to awaken Kundalini shakti. These can be practiced individually or in combination with each other.

AWAKENED IN CONNECTION WITH BIRTH

A few children are born with an already awake Kundalini. These children look at life very clearly, have a highly developed way of thinking and a very unusual way of looking at life. They often have no normal social relationship with their parents because they see them as "those who gave them life".

MANTRA

It is a powerful, gentle and risk-free method. However, it requires patience, time, discipline and regularity. Through mantra repetition and the vibration of sound, a wave of patterns is created that affects the mind. The physical, mental and emotional body is cleansed. It is important to focus the mantra on something by, for example, focusing on the tip of the nose or a chakra.

TAPASYA

It is a psychological procedure where you start a process that from the root eliminates bad habits that have created weakness and hinder development and willpower. Willpower is the core of tapasya. To enable the development and willpower, you want to curb the inner fire, live in celibacy, say no to lust, be restrained and, deny your own desires.

ASUHADHI - Using Herbs

This is the fastest and most effective method besides tantric initiation. It should not be confused with the use of drugs. Asuhadhi is a risky method that should only be done under the guidance of a guru.

RAJA YOGA

With Raja yoga, one merges the individual conscious-ness with the universal superconscious. This is done step by step with the help of concentration, meditation and the experience of unity with the absolute and highest self. When you focus and calm the mind, the sushum opens, which enables the rising of Kundalini. This is a mild method that is experienced to be difficult by many because it requires a lot of patience and discipline.

PRANAYAMA

Pranayamas are very powerful. If you are well prepared, live healthy, have a calm and safe place to practice breathing exercises, Kundalini can be awakened very quickly. Pranayamas strongly affect the body, creating heat while lowering the temperature in the inner body. Breathing changes the pattern of brain waves. It is important to cleanse the body with the help of shatkarmas before entering the process in order to better handle the rapid changes that come. Breathing is the link between Hatha and Kundalini yoga.

KRIYA YOGA

This is the simplest method for people living in the modern world. Here you do not have to confront the mind as in e.g. Raja yoga. People who are Sattvic may find it easy to awaken Kundalini through Raja yoga, but if you have a tumultuous mind that is constantly in motion, it only creates even more tension, guilt, complexes and sometimes even schizophrenia. When practicing Kriya yoga, Kundalini shakti is awakened slowly and metho-dically.

TANTRIC INITIATION

This method requires an understanding of what Shiva and Shakti stand for. You have to change your approach to passions and desires in life. Under the guidance of a guru, this is the fastest way to Kundalini awakening.

SHAKTIPAT

This method is performed by a guru. One experiences a temporary state of awakening - samadhi.

SURRENDER YOURSELF

This path means that one does not strive to awaken Kundalini Shakti. You let it happen when it happens and if it happens. It is believed that a strong enough will can arouse Kundalini.

PREPARATIONS

It is important to learn Kundalini yoga from a competent teacher so that one knows for sure that the process is going the right way. It is also important to be physically, mentally and emotionally prepared. Waking up Kundalini shakti can take time and you can count on it being a long process. However, there is nothing that says that Kundalini cannot wake up quickly. What really takes time is learning to keep the Kundalini alive.

*It is important that the sushumna is open, otherwise
Kundalini will rise along the ida or pingala which leads
to complications. The elements, chakras and nadis must
also be purified in order for Kundalini to flow freely.
This is done with the help of asanas, pranayamas and
Hatha yoga shatkarmas.*

*Surya namaskar and surya bheda pranayama cleanses
pingala nadi. Shatkarmas and pranayamas open up the
sushumna. You start by cleaning the elements with shat
karma. Then continue with asanas and pranayamas.
After that you can continue with mudras and bandhas.
Then you are ready to start with Kriya yoga.*

KARMA YOGA

*Karma yoga is a very important part of spiritual
development. Without Karma yoga, evolution will stop
no matter what method one chooses to follow. Karma
yoga prepares the mind. Positive and negative partners
become visible, consciousness is broadened and concentration is strengthened. Karma yoga is not a direct cause
of Kundalini awakening but an important part of the
process.*

DIFFERENT AWAKENINGS

*It is important to be able to distinguish between the
awakening of Kundalini, chakras and sushumna nadi. It
should also be possible to distinguish between an*

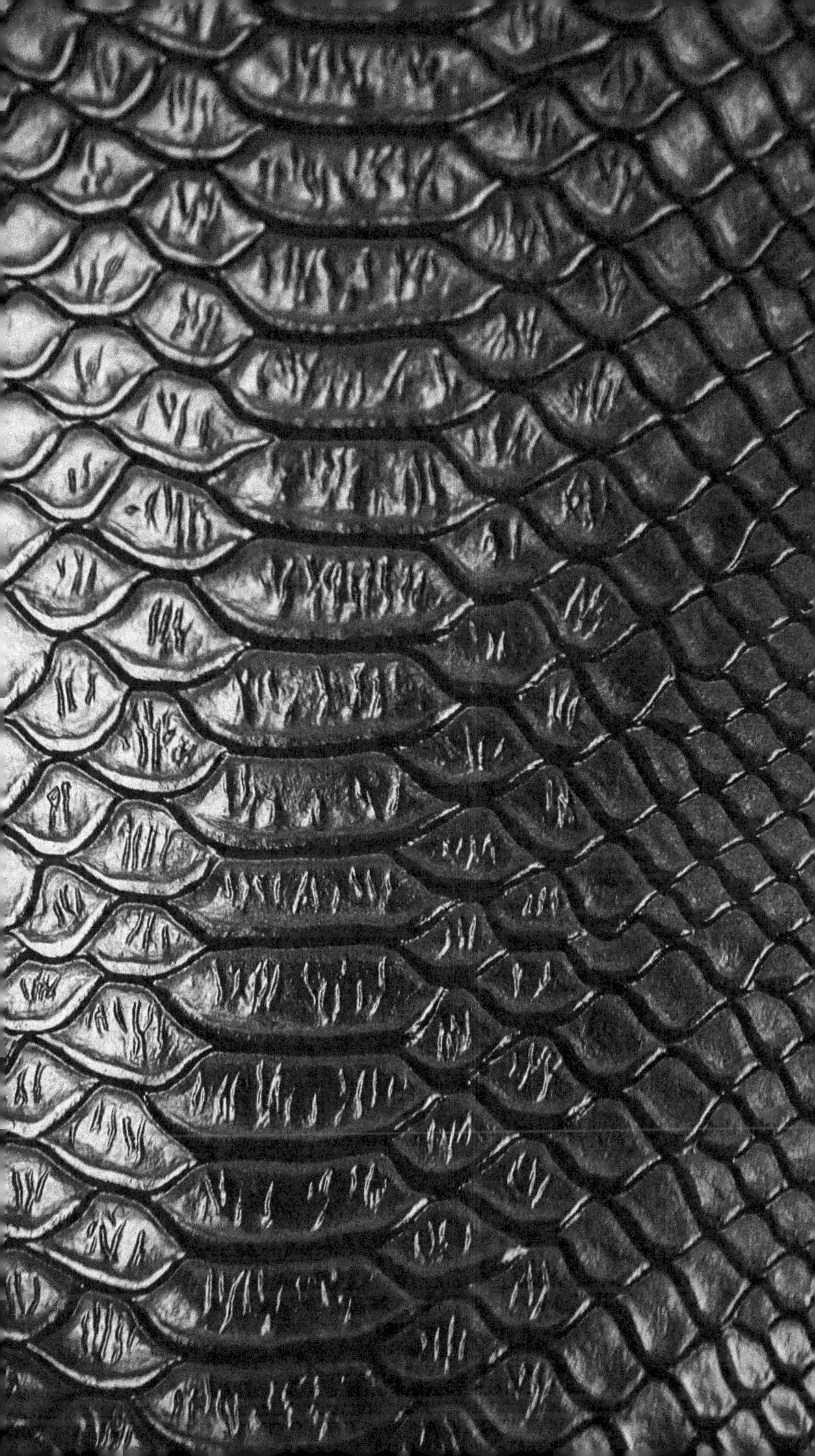

awakening between Mooladhara and Kundalini. The first step in awakening Kundalini shakti is to create harmony between ida and pingala nadi. The next step is to awaken the chakra system which leads to the sushumna opening and which allows for the Kundalini shakti to wake up.

When the process takes place in this order, you do not have to worry about negative consequences. If Kundalini instead wakes up before the sushumna is open, the energy will remain in the Mooladhara chakra and create sexual and neurotic disorders. Should any chakra not be open, Kundalini will get stuck in its path and create stagnation in development.

Harmony between ida and pingala nadi.

Pingala stands for the vital energy in the body. Ida stands for conscious energy. These two nadis control the two hemispheres of the brain, which in turn control all activity in the body. It is not really the awakening of these two that one strives for but a synchronization between them. As is well known, these control the body's temperature, digestion, hormonal secretion, the brain waves and the whole body's system. Bad food and lifestyle disturbs and creates an imbalance between them, which leads to physical and mental illness. Sus-

humna can only wake up when ida and pingala flow in harmony. Hatha yoga, pranayamas and Raja yoga are the best methods to create harmony between ida and pingala. Especially nadi shodhana.

Awaken the chakras.

All chakras must be balanced before the sushumna can wake up. Every little part of the body is connected to a chakra. Asanas open up the chakras in a gentle way. Sometimes a chakra can open quickly. Then feelings of fear, anxiety, passion, depression, etc. can emerge that have connections to previous experiences from previous lives.

Awaken the Sushumna.

It takes a lot of patience to awaken the sushumna nadi. You can expect to have experiences of a more intense nature than those that come when a chakra is awakened. These experiences are often completely illogical and strange. Hatha yoga and pranayamas are essential for awakening sushumna nadi.

KUNDALINI SINKS IN

After a rise, Kundalini will fall again. But the mind and consciousness will still be affected and changed. You get a higher state of consciousness. Our whole lives and our thoughts are affected. Emotions, body, and mind. Kundalini will be what characterizes life.

*When Shiva and Shakti become one in Sahasrara, one
experiences samadhi and silent parts of the brain wake
up. In this state, one is completely unaware of opposites,
man and woman, Shiva and Shakti - everything is one
and the same. During the experience of samadhi, Bindu
develops. Bindu means point and encompasses the
entire cosmos. It is the seat of human intelligence and
of all creation. After a while, the Bindu is divided into
two and the duality of Shiva and Shakti becomes reality
again.*

*Samadhi can be likened to the condition of an infant.
One does not know the difference between man and
woman and there is no physical or sexual difference.
When Shiva and Shakti return to the rough plane, down
to the Mooladhara chakra, they separate. Duality exists
in the mind in the world that consists of name and form
but not in samadhi.*

*When Kundalini sinks and you return to physical reali-
ty, you do it with a changed consciousness. You may live
your life just as before, with the same patterns, desires
and passions. What makes the difference is that you
observe life as if it were a spectacle.*

*You are in the theater of life just as before but as a spec-
tator. The changed consciousness is manifested through*

one. You are in contact with the parts of the brain that were previously silent. One is in contact with the knowledge, power and wisdom of the universe.

THE EXPERIENCE OF THE AWAKENING

A Kundalini rise can be likened to an explosion that takes you from one plane of consciousness to another plane of being. You travel through the borderland where perceptions, feelings and experiences change character. It is a journey between what you have experienced and the inexperienced.

The awakening takes place step by step and can take time. The preliminary awakening, and usually the first step, is the experience of light at bhrumadhya. This usually develops over a long period of time, in a very mild way and rarely creates any negative experiences. After a while, your appetite and need for sleep may decrease and your mind is still.

When the Kundalini rise finally takes place, it happens with power and sometimes you can experience things that are difficult to comprehend. One of the most common experiences is the feeling of "a current" along the spine. One can experience a burning sensation in Mooladhara and an energy flowing up and down along the sushumna. You can also hear sounds in the form of drums, bells, music, birds and flutes. You can also experience anger, passion and other repressed emotions that emerge. This usually passes within a few days. Some develop Siddhis which after a while also disappear.

You can lose your appetite for weeks, become depressed, lose interest in life and experience everything as very sad at the same time as the mind can become very mobile and creative. You might start writing poetry, creating music or some other art. This flattens out after a while and you land in your normal life and normal everyday life again. From the outside, everything looks like before, but you have an increased inner awareness and ability to observe. Headaches and insomnia can occur in some people when Kundalini wakes up.

It is easy to confuse the awakening of our chakras, nadis and sushumna with a Kundalini rise. When the chakra is opened, you get experiences that are usually pleasant and satisfying. They are rarely nasty or scary. When you get pleasant experiences during meditation or the kirtan or can feel the presence of your guru, it is a chakra awakening that takes place and not Kundalini.

When sushumna wakes up, you can experience the spine as shining or as a streak of light. You can also have sensual experiences that can seem very confusing and illogical. You can smell, hear screams or cry, feel warm or experience pain. Sometimes you can get disease symptoms and fever that doctors can not diagnose. When sushumna wakes up, you go through a form of depression, anorexia and loneliness. You begin to understand your inner being, your true nature. Materia is experienced as nothing and the body feels as if it were made of air or you can feel as if you are not a part of the body. You can communicate with your surroundings, trees, animals and water. You can start to anticipate things, but usually only boredom, accidents and disasters. You can feel reluctant to do work and it is good if at this stage you can be close to your guru to explain what is happening.

Fine visions and experiences are not always a sushumna or Kundalini awakening. It can still be chakras that open up, or experiences of samskaras and archetypes that emerge as a result of the sadhana that one follows. But to roughly sum it up, one can say that a Kundalini awakening always creates more abilities, Siddhis. If you slowly begin to understand language better, all of a sudden start to understand complicated things, all of a sudden become good at cooking, all of a sudden get a hearing in music, etc., then a gradual Kundalini awakening is taking place. If you experience temporary sensations and powerful light phenomena or visions, there may be other things that are connected to your chakras.

DIET

*When Kundalini is awakened, it is extremely important
to follow a proper diet as the food affects the mind and
human nature. During awakening, physical changes
occur in the body, mainly in the digestive system. The
body's internal temperature drops drastically and is
much lower compared to the outer body temperature.
Metabolism is slow and oxygen consumption decreases.
The food must therefore be easy to break down.*

*The best is cooked food. Crushed wheat, barley, lentils
and dal are preferred. Preferably in liquid form. Fatty
and heavy foods should be avoided and the amount of
protein should be kept to a minimum, as they strain the
liver and require a lot of energy to be able to be broken
down. When the mind undergoes a change, the liver
works hard.*

*It is good to increase the carbohydrates in the diet such
as rice, potatoes, wheat, and corn. These cause the internal body temperature to increase and do not require
much energy to digest.*

*Spices play a very important role for a Kundalini yogi.
Coriander, cumin, anise, black pepper, green pepper,
cayenne, mustard seeds, cardamom, cinnamon, etc.
support digestion. They store vital energy and support
the internal body temperature.*

KRIYA YOGA

Awakening Kundalini is difficult. Most yogic and religious paths are based on a lot of rules that require incredible self-discipline. Rishis in the tantric tradition developed a series of exercises that would be easy to follow and apply, regardless of lifestyle, beliefs or desires. Kriya yoga is seen as one of the most powerful of all tantric exercises and the path that is most suitable for modern man. The purpose of Kriya yoga is to open up the chakra system, purify the nadis and finally awaken the Kundalini shakti. Through the various kriyas, Kundalini is aroused gradually. It does not rise suddenly, which would be too difficult to handle.

Unlike other religions and yogic paths that often require strong mind control, in Kriya yoga one should not worry about the mind. Even if you can not concentrate or calm your mind, it does not matter - you develop anyway. Rishis in Kriya yoga believe that control of the mind is not necessary.

"Keep practicing and let the mind do what it does. In time, consciousness will reach the point where the mind no longer disturbs."

It is not always the fault of the mind that it is anxious or restless. Hormones, indigestion and a weak energy flow in the nervous system can be the cause. One should never blame the mind when it is restless, not even oneself. You are not stupid, bad, unclean or horrible even if you think evil thoughts. Everyone suffers from these, even the most peaceful and devoted. Trying to push back from the mind and thoughts and then see them come back again creates a division and in worst case causes mental illness. There is no good or evil mind. They are both one and the same. The mind is nothing but energy. Anger, passion, gratitude and joy are all different forms of the same energy. In Kriya yoga, one tries to utilize this energy without trying to silence or dampen it in any way.

In Kriya yoga, one does not try to concentrate or meditate. Mental control is not the purpose. The mind should flow freely and naturally. Kriya yoga is designed for individuals who find it difficult to sit still and stay focused for a long time. But - everyone should, whether you are tamasic, rajasic or sattvic, practice Hatha yoga as a preparation. A tamasic person needs Hatha yoga to awaken the mind and body. A person who is rajasic needs Hatha yoga to balance the vital and mental energies in the body and mind. A sattvic person needs Hatha yoga to make it easier to awaken Kundalini. In other words, Hatha yoga is for everyone and a preparation for

Kriya yoga. If you have practiced asanas, pranayamas, mudras and bandhas regularly for two years, you are usually ready for Kriya yoga.

There are many Kriyas but twenty of these are the most important and powerful. These twenty are divided into two groups. The first nine are done with open eyes and the remaining eleven are done with closed eyes.

In the first group of exercises, it is important that you really do not close your eyes even if you feel very relaxed and have an easy time turning your mind inward. You can blink, rest, take a break but do not close your eyes.

The first Kriyan is called Vipareeta Karani mudra. It is a method of creating a reverse process in the body. In Hatha Yoga Pradipika and the old tantric texts you can read about this process:

This nectar originates from the moon. As the sun consumes this nectar, the yogi ages. His body collapses and dies. Through regular practice, the yogi should try to reverse this process. The nectar flowing from the moon (Bindu) towards the sun (Manipura) should be returned to the higher centers. When the flow of amrit or nectar can be reversed, it will not be consumed by the sun. It will instead be assimilated by the body.

When the body has been cleansed with Hatha yoga,

pranayamas and a pure diet the nectar of the body is assimilated and one experiences a higher mental state. The mind is still and you see and hear everything much clearer.

It is said that one can influence and control the structure and energy of the body and thus evoke peace, dharana, dhyana or samadhi. The various exercises in Kriya yoga such as Vipareeta Karani mudra, Amrit Pan, Khechari mudra, Moola bandha, Maha mudra, and Maha Bheda mudra, regulate the nervous system. The prana in the body is harmonized and balanced. You achieve a state of peace and tranquility without having to fight against the mind. All this by creating a flow of unused and natural chemicals in the body. Amrit is one of them and through Khechari mudra you can make it flow. Khechari mudra is a simple but very important technique used in most kriyas. By turning the tongue upwards in the palate towards the nasal passage, specific glands and bandages are stimulated, resulting in the amrite starting to flow. One experiences shoonyata, a state of nothingness, being and awareness of everything. Body temperature drops and alpha waves begin to prevail. The mind is completely still.

When you have practiced yoga for a while and have reached the point where you have achieved concentra-

tion and a complete inner stillness in body, mind and soul but still feel that there is more to discover, you are ready for Kriya yoga. A calm mind, relaxed body and the right understanding are the results of a spiritual life, however, it is not the ultimate goal. The deeper meaning of yoga is to change the character of the experience, the pattern of the mind and its perception. Man's purpose in practicing yoga has been to expand the mind and release energy. It is tantra and the ultimate goal of Kriya yoga.

"THAT IS THE SIGN OF WISDOM: FREEDOM FROM DESIRE. ONLY FOOLS DESIRE. WISE PEOPLE LIVE AND LIVE JOYOUSLY, BUT WITHOUT DESIRE. EITHER YOU CAN DESIRE OR YOU CAN LIVE, YOU CAN NOT DO BOTH. IF YOU DESIRE, YOU POSTPONE LIVING; IF YOU LIVE, WHO BOTHERS ABOUT DESIRING? TODAY IS ENOUGH UNTO ITSELF."

THE CHAKRA SYSTEM

THE CHAKRA SYSTEM

In tantra and yoga, the lotus flower is used as a symbol for chakras. Man's spiritual development consists of three important phases: ignorance, striving, or, longing and enlightenment. In the same way, the lotus flower grows through three phases: clay, water and air. It grows in mud (ignorance), grows up through the water to the surface (striving and longing), and finally it comes up from the water and reaches the air and sunlight (enlightenment).

Each chakra is described as a lotus flower with a specific color and a number of petals. Each chakra consists of six different aspects:

1. Colour

2. Number of petals

3. Yantra (geometric shape)

4. Beeja mantra (sound / vibration)

5. Animal symbol (represents previous stages of evolution)

6. Higher / eternal being (represents the higher consciousness).

OUR CHAKRA

We have lots of chakras in our body but the most im-

portant ones are along our spine. There are also hidden so-called "Secret chakras".

The eight most important chakras in our body are:

MOOLADHARA CHAKRA

The root chakra is located at the base of the spine and is the chakra that vibrates with the lowest frequency, ie. the slowest of our seven chakras. Due to its frequency, its color is dark red and it has four petals. The element associated with this chakra is earth and stands for the most physical and down-to-earth with us.

SWADHISTHANA CHAKRA

The Swadhisthana chakra is located about two centimeters above the tailbone and is the center of our sexuality and reproductive ability. It has six petals, the color orange and its element is water.

MANIPURA CHAKRA

The Manipura chakra is located at the spine at the level of the solar plexus. It has ten petals and the color is yellow. The element fire controls Manipura and it is associated with will, worldly pursuit, ambition and career.

ANAHATA CHAKRA

The Anahata chakra is located in the spine behind the heart. It has twelve petals and the color is blue or green depending on the tradition you are studying. The element air dominates the chakra and controls our emotions and the relationship with other people. The Anahata chakra is also a symbol of love.

VISHUDDHI CHAKRA

Vishuddhi chakra is located in the neck and has sixteen petals. The color is violet and the element is space (ether). It controls our communication with the environment on different levels.

AJNA CHAKRA

The Ajna chakra is located in the middle of the head at the pineal gland and its contact area is the eyebrow center. It controls our paranormal abilities and Siddhis. Also called guru chakra or third eye. It is white in color and has two petals. It is associated with the mind, reason, intelligence and intuition.

BINDU VISARGA

According to tantra, Bindu visarga is a point located on the back of the head, where the Brahmins usually have their tuft of hair. It represents the crescent with a white drop, which stands for the manifestation of creation, such as consciousness.

SAHASRARA CHAKRA

The chakra is located just above the head and is purple /

red in color. It has a thousand petals and represents pure consciousness. When Kundalini shakti reaches Sahasrara chakra we become enlightened and according to yoga we enter nirvikalpa samadhi.

KSHETRAM

The exercises in Kundalini yoga usually focus on the trigger point of the chakra, which has its place at the spine. It can be difficult to experience in the beginning and many find it easier to focus on the point of contact on the front of the body called the chakra Kshetram. When we focus on a Kshetram, a sensation is created which then passes via the nerve pathways to the chakra and from there up to the brain. Mooladhara has no contact point, or, Kshetram.

GRANTHIS

We have three granthis (mental knots) in our physical body that are obstacles to Kundalini. These are called Brahma, Vishnu and Rudra. They describe the strength of the Maya, the ignorance and the attraction to material things. Level of consciousness. As an aspirant, one must overcome these obstacles in order for Kundalini to flow unhindered.

Brahma granthi has its place in the Mooladhara chakra and is associated with desire for material things, physical satisfaction and selfishness. It is also responsible for

tamas - negativity, lethargy and ignorance.
Vishnu granthi has its place at the Anahata chakra
and is associated with emotional desires, depending on
people and inner mental visions. It is linked to rajas and
has tendencies towards passion, ambition and determi-
nation.

Rudra granthi rules over the Ajna chakra. It is associa-
ted with the desire for Siddhis, mental phenomena and
the image of ourselves as individuals.

THE EVOLUTION THROUGH THE CHAKRANA

Human evolution as individuals and as a race is a jour-
ney through our chakras. Mooladhara is the base and
Sahasrara is the very goal or end of evolution.

In animals, Mooladhara is the highest chakra. It is their
Sahasrara. Until Mooladhara, evolution takes place by
itself, it is under the control of nature. When Kunda-
lini reaches Mooladhara, evolution no longer happens
automatically. Man is no longer subordinate to the laws
of nature. Man is aware of time and space. Man has
an ego, he can think, is aware that he is thinking and
he knows that he is aware that he is thinking. Without
the ego, there is no double consciousness. Animals do
not have a double consciousness. Man thus has a higher
consciousness and must therefore also work to develop

it. Therefore, it is said that Kundalini lies dormant in Mooladhara until it is awakened for further development.

Awakening Kundalini is a process. It may wake up to return to Mooladhara several times. When it finally reaches the Manipura chakra in a steady state, it will not turn again. What can happen is that it can get stuck in a chakra if there are blockages or if the sushumna is not open. Kundalini can remain in a chakra for several years or even a lifetime.

Before starting to practice Kundalini yoga, it is important to find out in which chakra Kundalini is located. The easiest way to do this is to focus on each chakra individually for fifteen minutes over a fifteen day period. You will notice which chakra is easiest to experience and stay focused on. Here is Kundalini shakti.

Awakening our chakras plays an important role in human evolution. It has nothing to do with mystery or anything occult. When the chakras are awakened, our consciousness and our mind change. This affects our daily lives as our mind is what controls how we act in different situations, relationships and emotions.

Today, many children are born with open chakras and

Kundalini. When these children grow up, they behave differently. Our modern society often sees these differences as something abnormal and the result is often mental health care or similar. Going through conflicts within family and work is a common phenomenon, but when the mind and consciousness begin to expand, one becomes extremely sensitive to everything that happens in the mind, family, colleagues and society. You can not overlook something that happens in life. It is not seen as normal by most people but it is a natural consequence of the chakra being awakened. Consciousness becomes very receptive when the frequency of the mind changes.

Love, devotion, charity, etc. are all expressions of a mind affected by the chakra in balance. This is the reason why so much emphasis is placed on awakening the Anahata chakra, or, the heart chakra. All chakras are of course important to open up and all have different qualities, but you can see that in most ancient scriptures put extra emphasis on awakening the Anahata, Ajna and Mooladhara chakra. When Anahata is awakened, we get a deeper relationship with our family and all individuals.

When the chakras are opened, the mind changes automatically. Values change and love and relationships change character. Disappointments and feelings of frustration are balanced, which leads to a better attitude towards ourselves and life.

PREPARATIONS FOR KRIYA YOGA

Kriya yoga is considered by many to be the most effective method of developing human consciousness. These exercises are said to be those that Shiva gave to his wife, Parvati. Kriyas are relatively simple and not too powerful for the average person to perform.

Before you start practicing Kriya yoga, it is important that you can feel the chakras in the body, both mentally and physically, and to be able to locate its Kshetram. One should also know two mental passages in the body "arohan" and "awarohan".

In order to develop in Kundalini yoga and in preparation for Kriya yoga, it is important to be well acquainted with the following techniques:

Vipareeta karani asana

Ujjayi pranayama

Siddhasana / Siddha yoni asana

Unmani mudra

Khechari mudra

Ajapa Japa

Utthanpadasana

Shambhavi mudra

Moola bandha

Nasikagra drishti

Uddiyana bandha

Jalandhara bandha

Bhadrasana

Padmasana

Shanmuki mudra

Varjoli / Sahajoli mudra

IDA AND PINGALA

Yogis have described that man has three main flows of energy in the body. Ida, pingala and sushumna nadi. These can be roughly translated as mind, body and spirit. Sushumna is the result of a balanced and harmonious flow between ida and pingala.

Nadis are flows of energy that move throughout our body. All the thousands of nadis that flow in the body are connected to the ida and pingala nadi that move along the spine. Every cell in our body, every organ, brain and mind are linked on a mental and physical level, which allows us to speak, think and act in a balanced and correct way. Ida and pingala nadi are the ones who control the balance between them. By affecting a part of the system, the whole system is affected. This is how asanas, pranayamas, meditation and the whole yogic system work. Yoga thus affects the entire system of nadis in our body.

Yogis and scientists have come to the same result, albeit with different ways of describing it. Man has two main modes through which he functions. The pattern of the brain is based on ida and pingala nadi, consciousness or knowledge, action or physical energy. We can see ida and pingala nadis functions in the three main parts of the nervous system.

Sensory-motor nervous system where all electrical activity in the body moves within two paths through the body. Into the brain (afferent), ida and out through the brain (efferent), pingala.

Autonomic nervous system which is divided into the outward, stress management, energy utilization, pingala dominant, sympathetic nervous system and inward, relaxed, energy saving, ida dominant parasympathetic nervous system.

Central nervous system which consists of the brain and spine and which controls the two preceding parts of the nervous system.

What the yogic techniques are based on is the knowledge of our nadis and chakras. The physical experience of these that you can also experience on a physical level through the different parts of the nervous system. The

The Chakranas
Colour, Number of Petals, Yantra
Action. Element & Bija mantra

Sahasrara chakra – I understand
Dark red, 1000 petals. Aum, Shiva

Ajna chakra
White, 2 Petals
Pyramid

Third Eye
I see
Moon Aum

Vishuddhi chakra
Purple 16 petals
Cirkel with Space

I talk
Space Element
Bija mantra Ham

Anahata chakra
Blue, 12 petals
Blue davidsstar

I love
Air element
Bija mantra Yam

Manipura chakra
Yellow, 10 petals
Red triangel

I do
Fire element
Bija mantra Ram

Swadhisthana ch.
Orange, 6 petals
Half moon

I feel
Water element
Bija mantra Vam

Mooladhara chakra – I am
Red 4 petals. Bija mantra Lam
Earth element, Yellow square

influence of the nervous system on our physical body describes the importance of balancing and harmonizing the flow between ida, pingala and sushumna nadi.

THE IMPORTANCE OF PREPARATION, EXERCISE AND NOT TAKING WATER OVER YOUR HEAD

As a beginner in yoga and full of desire and inspiration, it is easy to get water over your head. Yoga is a process in which the body and mind are prepared for more advanced techniques. It's like running. If you have run several marathons, you may need to run longer stretches to feel that the training gives something. This does not mean that you as a new runner do not get the benefits out of running three kilometers. This is exactly how yoga works.

When you have practiced Hatha yoga for a few years and feel comfortable in the positions with all the locks and postures and master the breathing exercises, you can move on with the most advanced tantric techniques. Then they will not feel too complicated and you will have a consciousness that allows you to enjoy the effects of your practice without it becoming too much. If something feels too complicated or difficult, go back one step instead. Everything comes to you when you are ready. Hurry slowly.

"You experience all the power in the
cosmos and on earth,
in yourself and around. Everything
you want is possible because all
power is yours!"

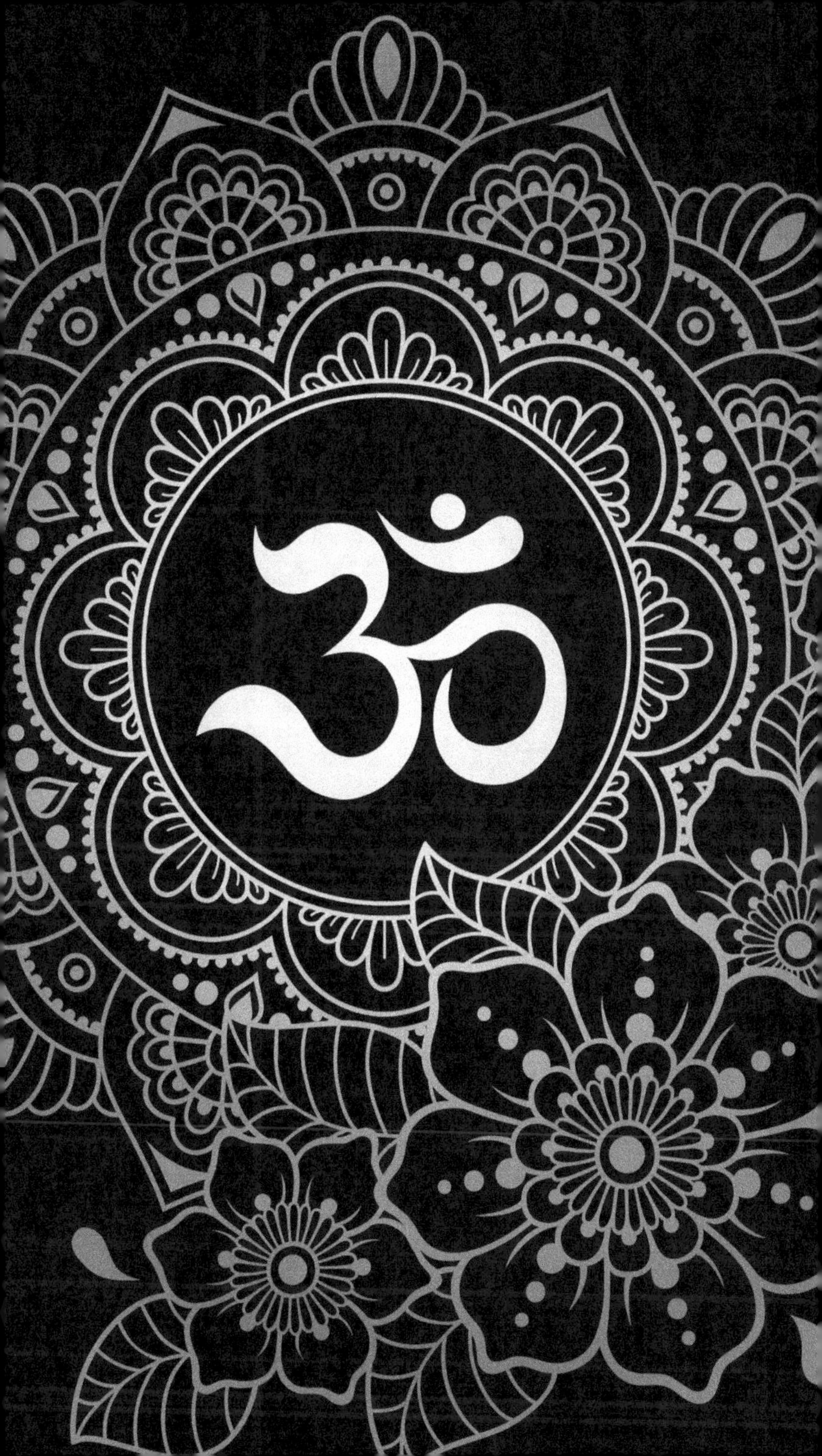

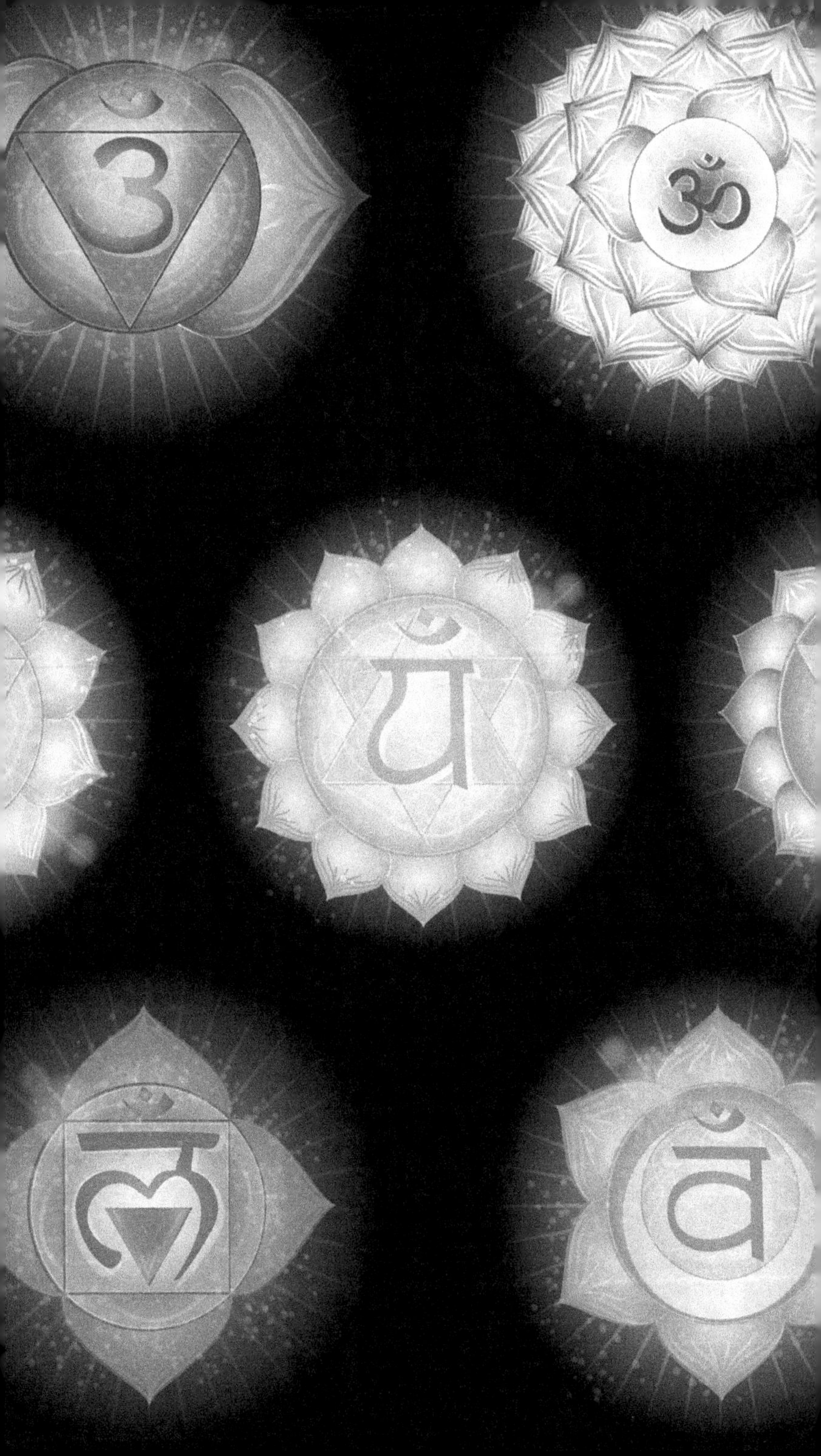

CHAKRANA
INDEX

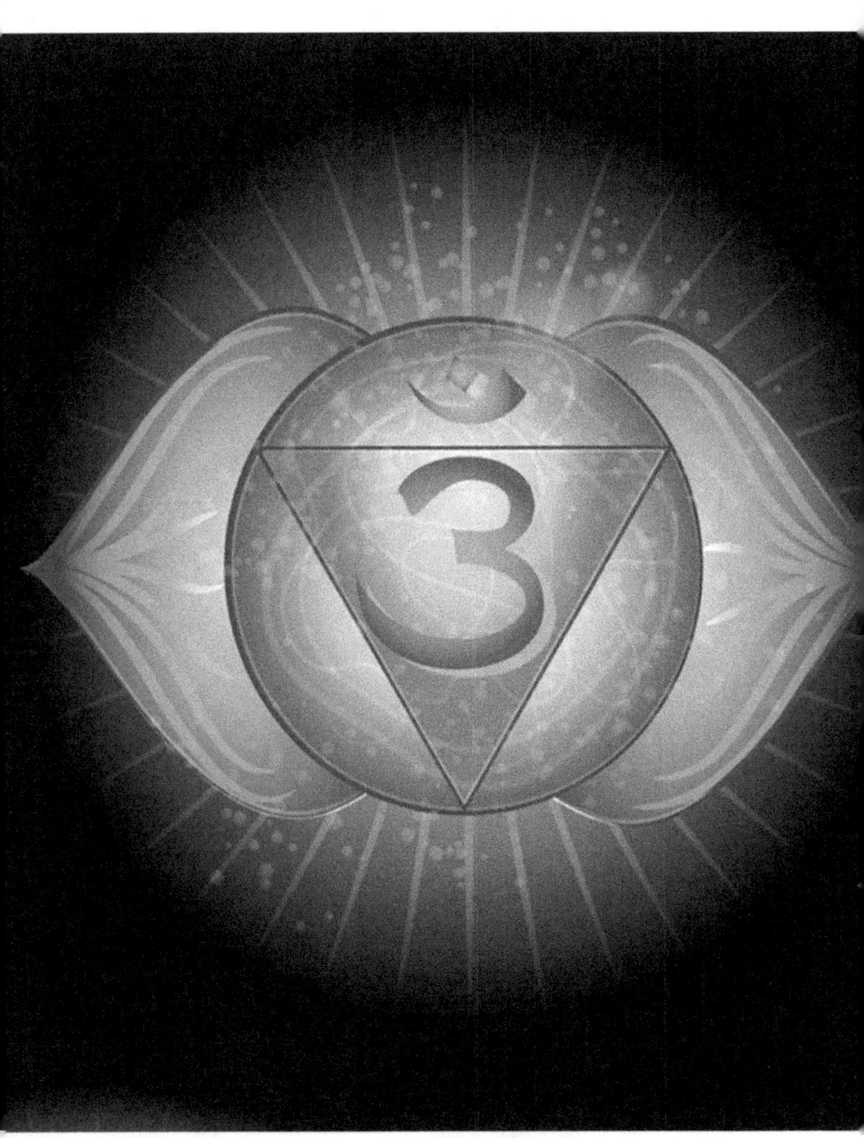

AJNA CHAKRA

ALSO CALLED THIRD EYE

TANMATRA *(sensory experience): Sense.*

JNANENDRIYA *(sense organ): Sense.*

KARMENDRIYA *(body of action): Sense.*

TATTWA *(element): Sense.*

BEJA MANTRA*: Om.*

TATTWA SYMBOL*: Picture of the mantra Om.*

YOGA TYPE*: Jnana, Raja and Mantra yoga (Sattvic).*

LOTUS (PADMA)*: White, silver or smoky with two petals.*

AJNA CHAKRA (third eye) is associated with the mind, reason, intelligence and intuition. It is also the center through which two people through the mind - on a deeper level, are in contact with each other. For example, the contact between guru (teacher / master) and student / disciple.

Direct concentration on the Ajna chakra is very difficult and therefore one focuses on tantra and yoga in the middle of the eyebrow center (which is in fact the Kshetram of the Ajna chakra). This point is called bhrumadhya (bhru- refers to eyebrows and -madhya refers to the center), and lies between the eyebrows at the place where Indian ladies put a red dot and Pandits and Brahmins put a mark. This eyebrow center can be touched by various techniques.

Ajna and Mooladhara chakras are closely related, and awakening in one of these helps to awaken the others. Ideally, Ajna should be awakened to some extent before Mooladhara in order to prepare the mind for all the hidden memories and impressions that come to the surface as we practice chakra awakening. But the awakening in Mooladhara will also help to further awaken Ajna. In fact, the best way to bring about the awakening of Ajna is Moola bandha and Ashwini mudra, which are specific to Mooladhara.

It should also be mentioned that the Ajna chakra and the pineal gland are one and the same. Just like the pituitary gland is the physical aspect of Sahasrara. The pituitary gland and the pineal gland are intimately connected to each other, as are the Ajna and Sahasrara. We can say that Ajna is the gateway to the Sahasrara chakra. If Ajna is awakened and works, then all experiences in Sahasrara happen as well.

The pineal gland acts as a lock for the pituitary gland. As long as the pineal gland is healthy, the pituitary gland works on a deeper, spiritual level. But for most of us, the pineal gland stops developing when we turn eight, nine or ten years old. This is when the pituitary gland begins to function and secrete various hormones that stimulate our sexual consciousness, our sensuality and worldly person. At this time, we started to lose touch with our spiritual heritage. However, through various yogic techniques, such as Trataka and Shambhavi mudra, it is possible to restore or maintain the health of the pineal gland. The pineal gland and Ajna chakra have a special significance in esoteric yoga and in tantra. It is the place where Siddhis (magical) abilities are manifested.

The "third eye" is a mysterious and esoteric concept that can refer to Ajna chakra in various spiritual traditions from East and West. It is also said to be a door that leads into inner worlds and stages of higher consciousness. In tantra and yoga, the "third eye" can symbolize enlightenment or the development of mental images with deeply spiritual or psychological meanings. The "third eye" is often associated with Siddhis such as revelations, clairvoyance (which also includes the ability to observe chakras and auras), divination, and out-of-body experiences. A person who is considered to have developed an ability to use his "third eye" is called a Siddha in yoga, and is referred to as a person who has developed Siddhis.

"THE PINEAL GLAND AND THE DMT MO-
LECULE - THE THIRD EYE ... THERE MAY
BE A WAY FOR THE BRAIN TO ACTUALLY
TAKE US TO A HIGHER PLANE OF EXISTEN-
CE, WHERE WE CAN UNDERSTAND THE
WORLD AND OUR RELATIONSHIPS TO
THINGS AND PEOPLE ON A DEEPER LEVEL
AND WHERE WE CAN ULTIMATELY CREATE
A DEEPER MEANING FOR OURSELVES AND
OUR WORLD. THERE IS A SPIRITUAL PART
OF THE BRAIN - IT IS A PART THAT WE CAN
ALL HAVE ACCESS TO AND IS SOMETHING
THAT WE ALL CAN ACCOMPLISH."

(ANDREW NEWBERG - BRAIN
RESEARCHER)

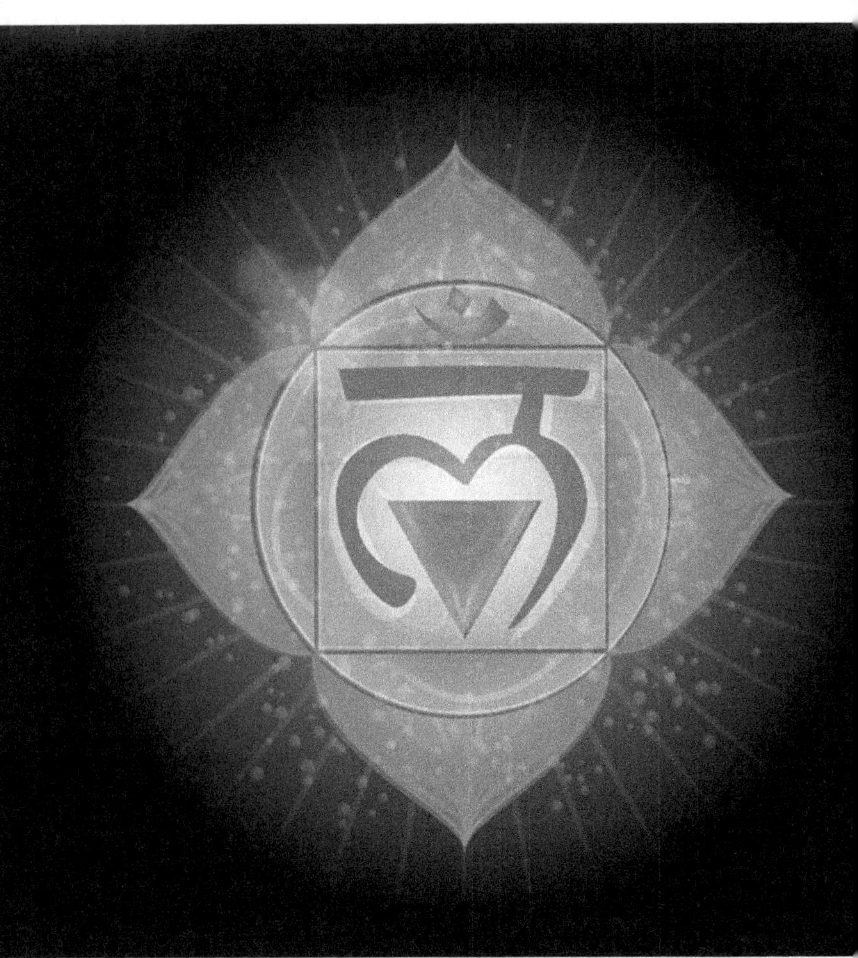

MOOLADHARA CHAKRA

TANMATRA *(sensory experience): Smell.*

JNANENDRIYA *(sense organ): Nose.*

KARMENDRIYA *(organ of action): Anus.*

TATTWA *(element): Prithvi (earth).*

BIJA MANTRA: *Lam.*

TATTWA SYMBOL: *Yellow square.*

ANIMALS: *Elephant.*

YOGA TYPE: *Tantra and Hatha yoga (counteracts tamas / inertia).*

LOTUS (PADMA): *Red lotus with four petals.*

MOOLADHARA CHAKRA

Moola means root. A triangular space in the middle of the body at a point between the genitals and anus for men and at the cervix for women. Mooladhara is associated with personal security in both thought and action. At this level, the individual focuses mainly on obtaining food and shelter and to secure his reproduction. She surrounds herself with material things, money, family and friends in order to create personal security.

In the middle of Mooladhara, one usually imagines a black swayambhu linga (a symbol of male power, Shiva). Around this, the serpent Kundalini (Shakti, the mother of all prana in the human body) winds three and a half turns - dozing in anticipation of its awakening, as it ascends through sushumna nadi to unite with Shiva in Sahasrara padma in the moment of enlightenment. This can only happen when the individual's spiritual development has reached the necessary maturity.

MOOLADHARAS IMPACT ON OUR DIFFERENT BODIES

IN ANNAMAYA KOSHA *(physical body).*
Reproductive organs, perineum, uterine tube.

IN PRANAMAYA KOSHA *(energy body).*
Apana vayu.

IN MANOMAYA KOSHA *(body of thought).*
Security, ownership, safety, survival.

MOOLADHARA IN DIFFERENT STAGES OF GUNAS

Creation and its energy consist of three gunas, fundamental properties or tendencies: Sattva, rajas and tamas. These three gunas act and react incessantly with each other. The world of phenomena is composed of different combinations of these three gunas. Tamas stands for inertia, rajas for movement and sattva for balance. When Mooladhara is in balance and sattvic, we are safe and secure in ourselves and in the world. When Mooladhara is out of balance and is tamasic, we experience boundless fear. We are in a deep psychosis. As the balance becomes more rajasic, our condition changes as shown below. By identifying one's state with the right degree of imbalance / balance in the various chakras, the yogi believes that he can alleviate and dissolve negative states.

TAMAS: *Horror.*

TAMAS / RAJAS: *Anxiety, worries.*

RAJAS / TAMAS: *Greed, self-confidence.*

RAJAS: *Collector.*

RAJAS / SATTVA: *Generosity.*

SATTVA / RAJAS: *Property for good cause.*

SATTVA: *Safe in the physical world.*

ENLIGHTENED: *Unity with the absolute*

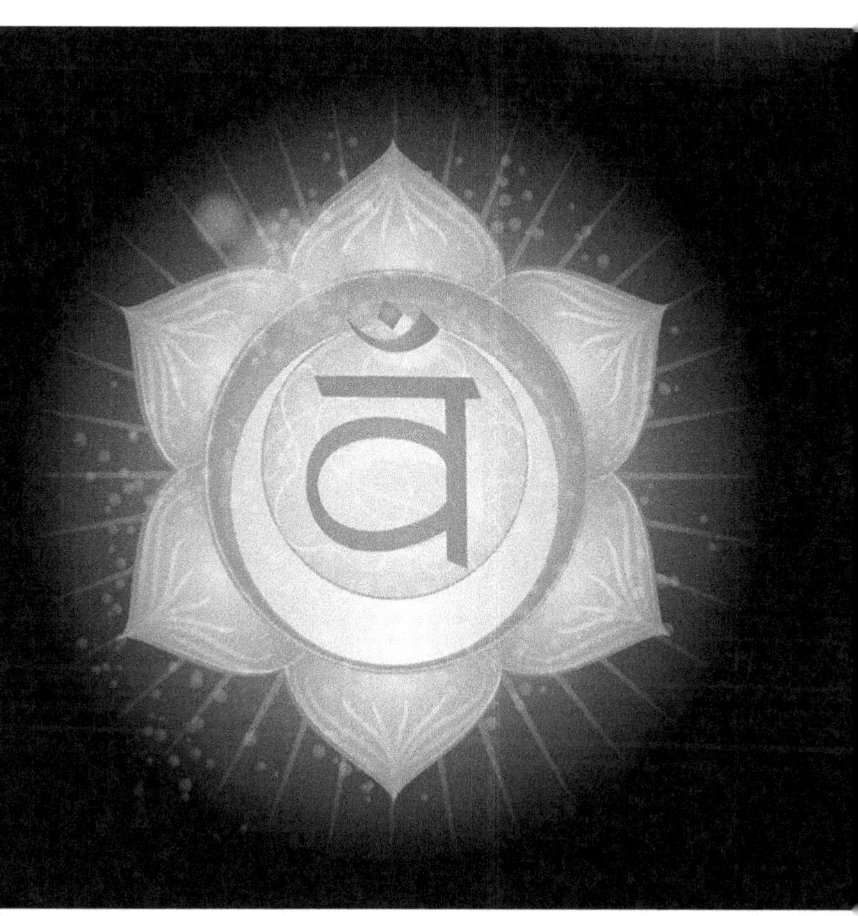

SWADHISTHANA CHAKRA

TANMATRA *(sensory experience): Taste.*

JNANENDRIYA *(sense organ): Tongue.*

KARMENDRIYA *(organ of action): Genitals.*

TATTWA *(element): Apas (water).*

BIJA MANTRA*: Vam.*

TATTWA SYMBOL*: White crescent.*

ANIMALS*: Crocodile.*

YOGA TYPE*: Tantra and Hatha yoga (counteracts tamas / inertia).*

LOTUS (PADMA)*: Orange lotus with six petals.*

SWADHISTHANA CHAKRA *(pleasure, lust)*
The chakra sits at the base of the spine just inside the lower tailbone and at the height of the genitals. Chakra is associated with sensory experiences. One strives to

achieve sensory enjoyment through e.g. food, drinks, sex, etc. You value everything in terms of the enjoyment you can thereby achieve. The difference from the Mooladhara chakra is that here we strive for the pleasure of the mind itself, rather than for satisfying the basic needs.

It is said that most people in the world primarily act and are motivated at this level. Swadhisthana chakra is also usually associated with the unconscious. It is said that coexistence - traces or patterns created in the unconscious of the experiences we make and the actions we perform, have their place in this chakra. Samskaras eventually form the basis of the individual's karma. Most of these cohabitants are displaced from consciousness or can be even repressed. Therefore, the Swadhisthana chakra is often associated with desires, urges, and fears over which we have no control.

THE IMPACT OF SWADHISTANS IN OUR DIFFE-RENT BODIES

ANNAMAYA KOSHA *(physical body): Genitals, urination.*

PRANAMAYA KOSHA *(energy body): Apana vayu.*

MANOMAYA KOSHA *(body of thought): Satisfaction, pleasure, sex (from pleasure to addiction).*

SWADHISTHANA IN DIFFERENT STAGES OF GUNAS

TAMAS: *Depression.*

TAMAS / RAJAS: *Bitterness, feeling of being rejected.*

RAJAS / TAMAS: *Desire, sexual exploitation.*

RAJAS: *Seeking pleasure, sexual conquests.*

RAJAS / SATTVA: *Humor, caring sexuality with love.*

SATTVA / RAJAS: *Happily satisfied.*

SATTVA: *Bubbly happy.*

ENLIGHTENED: *Ananda, happiness "bliss".*

MANIPURA CHAKRA

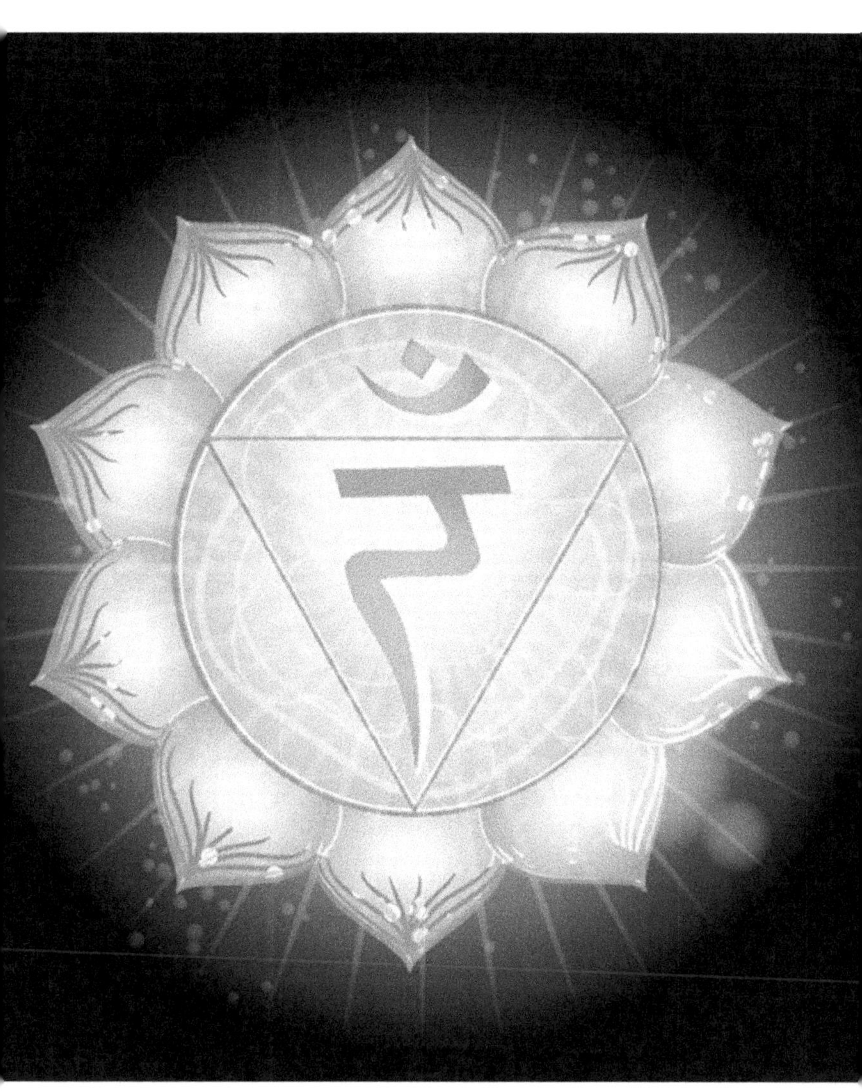

MANIPURA CHAKRA

TANMATRA *(sensory experience): Vision.*

JNANENDRIYA *(sensory organs): Eyes.*

KARMENDRIYA *(organ of action): Feet.*

TATTWA *(element): Agni (fire).*

BIJA MANTRA*: Ram.*

TATTWA SYMBOL*: Red inverted triangle.*

ANIMALS*: Aries.*

YOGA TYPE*: Karma yoga (counteracts rajas / mobility).*

LOTUS (PADMA)*: Yellow lotus with ten petals.*

MANIPURA *(seat of the jewel)*
The chakra is located in the spine at the level of the navel. It is associated with will, worldly pursuit, ambition and career. From the energy of manipulation, man grows as a social and self-conscious being. She cultivates material desires, such as owning and mastering, power,

prestige and usefulness. But also selflessness, social balance and prosperity.

Manipuras energy is outward and active, a vital energy that provides the power to act and the power to change oneself and one's surroundings. Sometimes this happens with a selfish attitude where other people are seen as a means to achieve their own ambition, but here also the first expressions of a growing self-awareness begin to take shape in man. The ego is still dominant but the first traces of a genuine, spiritual pursuit are manifested at this level. One begins to seriously question one's existence and one's motives.

THE IMPACT OF MANIPURAS IN OUR DIFFERENT BODIES

ANNAMAYA KOSHA *(physical body): Solar Plexus, digestion.*

PRANAMAYA KOSHA *(energy body): Samana vayu.*

MANOMAYA KOSHA *(body of thought): Power, action, self-confidence and striving.*

MANIPURA IN DIFFERENT STAGES OF GUNAS

TAMAS: *Inability to act.*

TAMAS / RAJAS: *Guilt over non-actions, low self-esteem.*

RAJAS / TAMAS: *Frustration over one's own inability.*

RAJAS: *Active, brave.*

RAJAS / SATTVA: *Anxious, ready to act.*

SATTVA / RAJAS: *Karma yoga at an intermediate level.*

SATTVA: *Things happen as if by miracle.*

ENLIGHTENED: *Omnipotent.*

"AND WHEN LOVE GOES DEEPER,
FEAR DISAPPEARS.

LOVE IS THE LIGHT, FEAR IS DARKNESS."

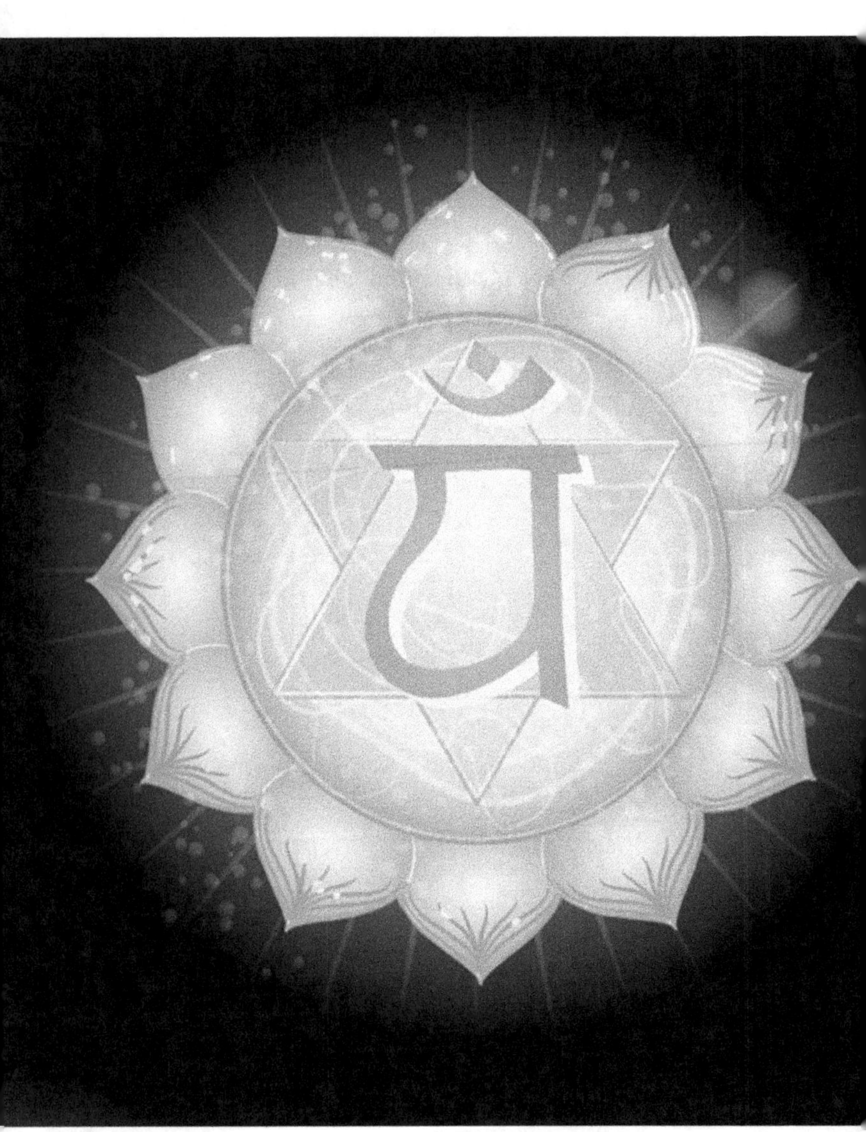

ANAHATA CHAKRA

TANMATRA *(sensory experience): Feeling.*

JNANENDRIYA *(sense organ): Skin.*

KARMENDRIYA *(body of action): Hands.*

TATTWA *(element): Vayu (air).*

BIJA MANTRA*: Yam.*

TATTWA SYMBOL*: Blue hexagram.*

ANIMALS*: Black antelope.*

YOGA TYPE*: Bhakti and Karma yoga (counteracts rajas / mobility).*

LOTUS (PADMA)*: Blue or green lotus with twelve petals.*

ANAHATA (unspoken "sound", the origin of all mant-ras). Anahata sits in the spine at the height of the heart. Its energy is associated with love, hate, joy and sorrow as well as with the beauty experience. Chakra is strongly associated with our relationships with others around us. At this level, the individual often begins to love eve-

*rything and everyone unconditionally. You learn
to ignore the faults and shortcomings of others and
take them for what they are. Anahata also stands for
aesthetic discernment and artistic creation. The energy
is expressed here in the form of creativity regardless of
which area you are active in. At this level, man leaves
the material world to cultivate higher values.*

THE INFLUENCE OF ANAHATAS IN OUR DIFFERENT BODIES

ANNAMAYA KOSHA *(physical body): Heart, lungs.*

PRANAMAYA KOSHA *(energy body): Vyana vayu.*

MANOMAYA KOSHA *(body of thought): Love, compassion, acceptance and tolerance.*

ANAHATHA IN DIFFERENT STAGES OF GUNAS

TAMAS: *Apathy.*

TAMAS / RAJAS: *Fraud, treason.*

RAJAS / TAMAS: *Avoid intimacy.*

RAJAS: *Love under certain conditions.*

RAJAS / SATTVA: *Care about others.*

SATTVA / RAJAS: *Love and compassion.*

SATTVA: *Is love.*

ENLIGHTENED: *Cosmic love.*

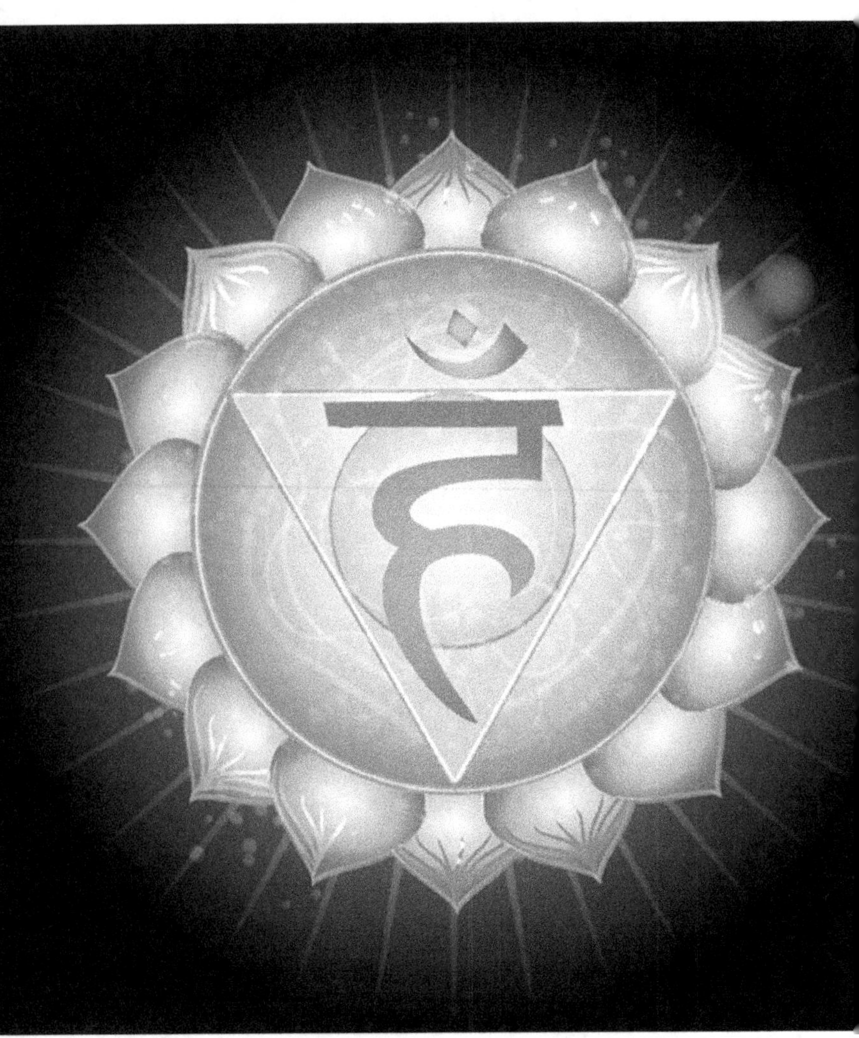

VISHUDDHI CHAKRA

TANMATRA *(sensory experience): Sound.*

JNANENDRIYA *(sensory organs): Ears.*

KARMENDRIYA *(body of action): Body of speech.*

TATTWA *(element): Akasha (space).*

BIJA MANTRA*: Ham.*

TATTWA SYMBOL*: White and black circle.*

ANIMALS*: White elephant.*

YOGA TYPE*: Jnana, Raja and Mantra yoga (sattvic)*

LOTUS (PADMA)*: Violet lotus with sixteen petals.*

VISHUDDHI *(purity).*
The chakra sits in the neck behind the larynx and is associated with an attitude of independence (vairagya), where both pleasant and unpleasant aspects of human life are seen and accepted as rewarding experiences. The world appears as a place full of harmony and perfection. Everything you experience, good or bad, is seen as part

of a whole that helps to remove personal problems, locks and limitations and raise the level of consciousness. This attitude leads to discernment (viveka).

Vishuddhi is also associated with expression, communication in general and the spoken word in particular.

THE IMPACT OF VISHUDDHI IN OUR DIFFERENT BODIES

ANNAMAYA KOSHA *(physical body): The thyroid gland, parathyroid gland, trachea and esophagus.*

PRANAMAYA KOSHA *(energy body): Udana vayu.*

MANOMAYA KOSHA *(body of thought): Communication.*

VISHUDDHI IN DIFFERENT STAGES OF GUNAS

TAMAS: *Isolated.*

TAMAS / RAJAS: *Limited contact / communication.*

RAJAS / TAMAS: *Complaining / whining.*

RAJAS: *Pretty good communicator.*

RAJAS / SATTVA: *Eloquent.*

SATTVA / RAJAS: *Persuader, non-violent communi-cation.*

SATTVA: *True communication.*

ENLIGHTENED: *Cosmic communication.*

BINDU VISARGA

Bindu visarga is located on top of the back of the head. Many claim that one can not find Bindu in the physical body but that it can only be experienced via nada, ie. via its vibration or sound. It is not really a chakra in the ordinary sense.

Through techniques like Moorcha pranayama and Vaj-roli / Sahajoli mudra we can develop the experience of nada and through techniques like Bhramari pranayama and Shanmukhi mudra we can follow nada to its source - Bindu.

There is a close relationship between the Swadhisthana chakra and the Bindu. This is because Bindu is the point where the vibration and sound of the individual crea-tion is first manifested, and Swadhisthana is the center of creation in the form of sexual reproduction. Through Swadhisthana, our physical desire for union with the cosmic consciousness is expressed. Sperm and menstru-ation are physical expressions of the drops of amrit - the nectar drops of creation or secretions that drip from the Bindu and are burned in the Manipura chakra via the Vishuddhi chakra. The drops that control the creation process and the body's aging.

It is commonly believed that there is no Kshetram - contact point for Bindu visarga.

SAHASRARA CHAKRA

The chakra is located just above the head and is purple / red in color. It has a thousand petals and represents pure consciousness. When Kundalini shakti reaches Sahasrara chakra we become enlightened and according to yoga we enter Nirvikalpa samadhi.

The function of the Sahasrara is to provide us with other levels of consciousness, which may make us realize that "we are one" and that "everything is one". It is through the crown chakra that we experience union with God and with the supernatural. The Crown Chakra is what is called "pure consciousness".

When one reaches the higher level of consciousness in this chakra, all thinking is released. Here lay the answers to all our questions, the absolute truth that we all dream of getting answers to, and where we find total freedom - We become enlightened.